The Great Pendulum Book

The
Great
Pendulum Book

Petra
Sonnenberg

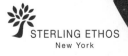

STERLING ETHOS
New York

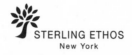

STERLING ETHOS
New York

An Imprint of Sterling Publishing
1166 Avenue of the Americas
New York, NY 10036

This edition published in 2015 by Sterling Publishing Co., Inc.

Originally published under the title Pendelen van A tot Z
by Uitgeverij Schors, Amsterdam, Netherlands

Text © 1998 by Uitgeverij Schors

Translation © 2003 by Sterling Publishing Co., Inc.

Translation by Nicole Franke and Daniel Shea

ISBN 978-1-4549-1717-5

Distributed in Canada by Sterling Publishing
c/o Canadian Manda Group, 664 Annette Street
Toronto, Ontario, Canada M6S 2C8
Distributed in the United Kingdom by GMC Distribution Services
Castle Place, 166 High Street, Lewes, East Sussex, England BN7 1XU
Distributed in Australia by Capricorn Link (Australia) Pty. Ltd.
P.O. Box 704, Windsor, NSW 2756, Australia

For information about custom editions, special sales, and premium and corporate purchases,
please contact Sterling Special Sales at 800-805-5489 or specialsales@sterlingpublishing.com.

Manufactured in Canada

2 4 6 8 10 9 7 5 3 1

www.sterlingpublishing.com

Contents

Overview of the Pendulum Charts

Inner Growth and Spirituality

GUIDING PRINCIPLE AND INSPIRATION

ORACLE AND GUIDE

TAROT

RUNES

Environment

Foreword

The pendulum has become more and more popular in recent years. It owes this popularity to its very clear answers to complicated and difficult questions. It provides the kinds of answers that are often hard to come by, because the questions can become too complex if we give them much thought.

Using the pendulum is a relatively new technique. The more famous divining rod—or dowsing rod—is basically its predecessor and has been used for a much longer period of time, but both function with the same forces and techniques. Work with the pendulum, as we know it today, is of a later date than is generally assumed. Although dozens of books have been published about it in the past decades and much research has been done, the operation of the pendulum has remained rather traditional, if not conservative—in any case, it has not been what you might call innovative.

This lasted until the end of the 70s when the Swiss Willy Kowa did some research for the magazine *Schweizerische Zeitschrift für Radiästhesi*. He had the idea of categorizing the questions that people ask when using the pendulum and putting them into visual form. Since then many people, among them I myself, have followed his example.

The idea was to pose a short, direct question on a certain topic and sum up a specific number of answers in a kind of chart, so that question and answer are visually coupled with one another. The result of this idea was that the possibilities for operating the pendulum increased tremendously. In contrast to earlier times, when the pendulum was a kind of modern divining rod, the experienced pendulum user today can access far more information quickly, and will work with at least three different kinds of pendulums.

No longer used exclusively to complement other esoteric techniques, the pendulum has taken up an important place as a tool for retrieving information in psychology, medicine, and even in very "worldly" matters, such as street construction.

Petra Sonnenberg has succeeded in putting together a pendulum guide that at last releases the pendulum from its occult stigma. Here she has arranged 125 pendulum charts according to their topic and supplied a clearly laid out index. She explains rationally and clearly in several chapters what exactly a pendulum is, what "pendulum work" means, and how to integrate it into our daily life as an aid in solving problems of the most diverse kinds.

Anyone who works with the pendulum or is interested in exploring it will discover in this book a refreshing complement to already existing literature on this topic, placing this technique in an entirely new light. I am convinced that it will, over the years, become one of the standard texts about work with the pendulum.

I wish you all great joy with this innovative book.

D. Jurriaanse
Terracino, 1998

Introduction

Some history

The posing of questions to the pendulum has already been practiced for a long time and still attracts a lot of people today. It has been used by our ancestors in order to make supposedly "invisible" things visible. It enables us to receive information that is not accessible by any other means.

Always surrounded by an air of mystery, the practice of divining with the pendulum was not without danger. In the Middle Ages it was, for instance, connected with witchcraft and punishable by death. Less threateningly, it was labeled as "nonsense" and brushed aside as an occupation of people who were allegedly "not from this planet."

What exactly is this pendulum work? Is it a mysterious ritual that can only be performed by the initiated? Is it a kind of "thought reading"? Or is it simply the picking up of certain energies?

All living beings—humans, animals, plants, and even crystals, minerals, and so on—are surrounded by an aura of radiation that contains a certain kind of information. Both the pendulum and the divining rod pick up this radiation and localize it. This process is called "radiesthesy"—coming from radius (Latin: "ray") and aestheses (Greek: "to perceive"); thus, the term simply means "to perceive radiation." Radiesthesy was (and is) not only practiced for finding various "good" energies and energy sources but also to defend against harmful influences; in these cases, the pendulum and divining rod serve as instruments.

How long the pendulum and the divining rod have been used is not known with any precision. It is also uncertain where they were applied for the very first time. Both in regard to time and place, sources vary tremendously. In North Africa, for instance, diviners can be recognized in cave paintings that date back to about the year 6000 b.c.e. Other sources lead us to China where a famous diviner was supposed to have lived 2000 years before Christ. Discoveries from the Roman period in Europe (1st century c.e.) reveal the operation of the pendulum. Diviners or "oscillators" are illustrated in woodcuts that have been preserved from the Middle Ages.

Generally, it is assumed that the divining rod has probably been used for a much longer period of time than the actual pendulum, and that the development and application of the pendulum developed out of work with the divining rod.

What exactly is measured with these instruments?

The divining rod is usually produced from natural material, such as, for example, a forked branch from the hazelnut bush. It was—and still is—used in the search for earth currents, water, minerals, and other energy sources: in the so-called "walking with the dowsing rod," the diviner holds the forked branch horizontally with both hands, "stem" pointing forward. When the branch picks up the radiation that an energy source radiates, the end of the branch moves and "kicks out." When it does that, the energy source can be located precisely.

The choosing of a suitable hazelnut branch is not a simple matter. Both the quality of the wood and the shape of the branch have to meet certain requirements. Dowsing rods are therefore random and unique. Since their beginning, as time went by, divining rods were also made from other conductive materials (such as, for example, copper), which are equally suitable, yet easier to obtain. Different shapes are also used.

Due to its size and shape, the divining rod is well suited for use in the open country and for things that are linked to sowing, planting, cutting, and harvesting. It is also used in the search for an ideal location for new cultivation, a location that has a desirable radiation in the soil.

The smaller measuring instrument—the pendulum—was developed for use in a more refined application of radiesthesy. It is especially useful for measuring the radiation that surrounds us.

The invisible information that lies "hidden" in this radiation can help us a great deal in our search for answers to questions of the most varied kinds. It is also helpful in discovering the causes of different phenomena that have been inexplicable up to this point.

The diviner suspends the pendulum by a thread or on a chain over the place or object about which he or she would like to learn more. The pendulum picks up the radiation (energy) of this place or object, which the diviner can then perceive clearly.

He or she can "feel" this energy in the pendulum, and, if there is sufficient energy, the pendulum will begin to swing noticeably.

Whenever this phenomenon is linked to a question and with an often-used aid—the so-called pendulum chart—the information becomes clearly identifiable. The answer can be read from the pendulum chart or from individual pendulum gyrations ("yes" or "no"). The questioner finds an answer with the help of the pendulum, which makes the useful piece of information "visible."

Research

Science has been occupying itself for a very long time with the function and meaning of pendulum movements, which are also called "oscillations."

At the beginning of the 20th century, associations were founded in England and America (which were sometimes secret) that occupied themselves with oscillating and walking with the dowsing rod, and tried to explain these phenomena. After some time—once the shroud of secrecy around the pendulum was lifted—a special "school" was even founded in which classes were taught dealing with the work of the dowsing rod and the pendulum. Many theories were established, and just as many textbooks were written, but there was still disagreement about it.

Even the famous scientist Galileo researched the duration of the oscillations of the pendulum and its different dependencies. However, his research focused primarily on gravity (the force of attraction of the earth). As measuring instruments, he used pendulums made from different materials. A pendulum or a weight on a thread tends to level out in a certain direction: namely the point at which the force of attraction of the earth is greatest. It turned out that the oscillating time of different pendulums varied in length. He concluded from this that gravity has an equally strong effect on different substances.

Most recent scientific laboratory experiments have shown that there must indeed be a certain kind of energy that sets the pendulum in motion and that the oscillations of the pendulum are not based on pure chance. Many believed that the energy is Extra Sensory Perceptions (ESP). Experiments lent credibility to the idea that some people are more receptive to these kinds of energies than others. But what precisely the energies were and how they influenced the pendulum could not be clarified.

All modern experiments and developments pointed to the same conclusion: when working with the pendulum, other criteria also play a role, besides the force of attraction of the earth alone; a force, unknown up to this point, is somehow involved.

Today's Application

The pendulum is used today primarily for picking up the cosmic radiation that surrounds us. It enables the skillful practitioner to convert this radiation into information that is helpful for us. The focus, however, does not lie exclusively on practical matters, such as the search for energy sources and earthly radiation, but also on a personal and spiritual level as well, such as the discovery of disturbances in our physical or spiritual balance, and the answering of important personal questions. In short, it can deal with diverse matters that can aid us in our individual lives and spiritual evolvement.

Basically, working the pendulum is nothing but the making visible answers to the questions of life with the help of our unconscious. The pendulum provides an answer that is more than the rational consideration of carefully thought-through arguments. It reveals to us things that lie much more deeply hidden in our minds and thus uncovers the true character of both question and answer. This insight can help us to obtain a better understanding of ourselves and thus enable us to make wiser decisions.

As question and answer are set free from superfluous details and trimmings, we are confronted with the "bare facts." In this way, it is also possible to disassemble complex situations into smaller parts that are easier to deal with. A difficult question can now be answered step-by-step without our becoming wrapped up in irrelevant matters that cloud the true picture lying at the root.

Therefore, the pendulum can give us reliable advice when we come to a crossroads, by revealing our possibilities and talents, for instance, or making visible deeply anchored considerations and desires. With this clarity, we can make better choices.

Also, in other important areas of our life, the pendulum can play an important role. For instance, we can use it to determine what may have been inexplicable causes of disease, as well as what possibilities are open to us when facing the choice of alternative medical treatments or alternative medications. And, in the case of troublesome sufferings that cannot be cured with medical treatment, the pendulum can provide good service. The factors that lie at the root of the problem can be successfully analyzed step-by-step. We are then confronted with the true causes—and even possibly hidden motives—that are the underlying reason that we do not change (or perhaps do not want to change) a particular situation.

Over the years, the pendulum has definitely been filling an important role of reliable advisor when searching for alternative solutions and the fostering of personal, spiritual development. We use it not only to help ourselves, but also to help others as we simplify this process and further its applications.

In this book, we will occupy ourselves above all with the idea that the pendulum really works. Exactly how it works, we will leave with all clear conscience to the work of others.

Getting to Know
the Pendulum

Before we begin working with the pendulum, it will help us to learn more about it. What is a pendulum? From what kind of material can a pendulum be produced? How can we apply these various materials? How large or small is a pendulum allowed to be? As we shall discover, pendulums are very diverse.

What does a pendulum look like?

A pendulum is, simply expressed, a weight (of not too great a size) that hangs on a (not too long) piece of thread or on a chain. The diviner holds the pendulum between thumb and index finger so that the pendulum can move unhindered (swinging or spinning out) over an object that is to be questioned.

The most important feature of this weight on a string is its oscillation in the direction of the greatest force of attraction. And it will become clear that diverse factors can influence the mobility and the effects of the pendulum. (At this time, we are focusing on the pendulum and not on conditions that have to do with the environment).

The following factors can exert an influence in different ways and manners. For instance:

Material of the pendulum:	specific weight
	form and size
	conductivity or influence
Thread or chain on pendulum:	material and structure
	shape and length

The Material of the Pendulum

Specific Weight

The material of which the pendulum is made influences the movement of the pendulum in a number of ways. Each material has, for instance, a specific weight: the heavier the material, the slower the oscillation of the pendulum. Its mobility is thus dependent upon the influence that gravity exerts on the material.

Form

When choosing the pendulum, we are not bound to a single shape. It can vary from a bowl down to a small cylinder; it can even be a combination of different shapes. When choosing the shape of the pendulum that is right for you, let yourself be guided by its shape ("Does the shape of the pendulum appeal to me or not?") or the usefulness of its shape. It is important that the pendulum has a clearly pointed edge that can indicate the requested information—the "answer." A clearly pointed edge at the lower side of a (spherical or conical) pendulum is, for instance, workable, as is a (narrow) cylindrical pendulum that comes to a point at the bottom. The clearer the point or the pointed edge, the more exact the information that can be read.

The choice of material also influences the shape: precious metals can be poured into almost any desired or suitable mold: spherical or cylindrical pendulums with a clear pointed edge;

oblong or conical pendulums, one side of which has a pointed edge; pendulums that can be disassembled so that the shape and size of the pendulum can be made bigger or smaller); or pendulums that can be filled, for instance, with the dust of precious stones, essential oils, or certain herbs (herbal essences).

Pendulums made from precious stones can find special uses due to their facets or the original shape of the stone or crystal.

Size

The size of the pendulum will be influenced by the material used. The heavier the material, the smaller the pendulum: thus, the lighter the material (for example, wood), the more the shape needs to be taken into consideration.

Conductivity or Influence

In addition, the conductivity of the material is important. Quartz is, for example, a better conductor than brass. The better the material conducts, the clearer the information the user has to read. It is, however, worth mentioning that this "conductivity" is a very personal thing. Some diviners, for example, prefer to work with crystals or precious stones, while others prefer precious metals or alloys of various metals. If you try several pendulums of various materials, you will very soon notice which kind of material works best for you.

There are, however, some areas in which the material of the pendulum can influence its movement, especially when "natural" materials are used.

EXAMPLE I

"Does this rose quartz fit the constellation of Taurus"? (Answer: "yes" or "no.")

A pendulum made of rock crystal (a natural material) could give, when questioning a certain kind of precious stone, an unexpected or imprecise answer—or even no answer at all—to the question posed. In this case, even a clearly negative answer cannot be excluded, although rose quartz is a stone that is especially ascribed to the constellation of Taurus!

Why would the pendulum give a wrong answer in this case? Take into consideration that a pendulum made of a natural material has its own special characteristics. Rock crystal is, for instance, transparent, almost colorless, and naturally cool (crystal derives from the Greek word *krystallos*, which means ice). Rock crystal has a cleansing and cooling effect and is, so-to-speak, "unique" as a transmitter of "divine light." The constellation Capricorn is ascribed to it.

For this reason, it's no surprise that a pendulum made of rock crystal does not know what to do with a piece of rose quartz! The characteristics of rose quartz are diametrically opposed to those of rock crystal. Rose quartz is a warm light pink and has a calming, loving, and harmonizing effect. It is a "social" stone, and thus is assigned to the constellations of Taurus and Libra (both ruled by Venus).

In this way, the characteristics of certain materials can influence one another and lead to "wrong" answers with certain questions. In such a situation, it is better to use a pendulum that is made from an entirely different material than the object to be questioned. In this case, a pendulum made from nickel or brass would be quite suitable for the question.

EXAMPLE 2

"Can I use a wooden pendulum for the localization of possible causes of illnesses"? (Answer: "yes" or "no.")

This should work out without any problems; we can choose from many different kinds of wood. However, due to its grounding features, and although wood is in general neutral, a wooden pendulum will not conduct radiation as well as a pendulum made from brass, which is a good conductor. Here also a pendulum made from brass will probably lead to a more accurate result.

It is also important to know that some kinds of wood have a healing effect, such as, for example, sandalwood and cedar; they are, due to their special healing features, excellent to use in amulets. However, start by questioning—with a pendulum made from brass or copper—specifically what kind of harm this amulet will protect against!

Example 3

"Can I use a pendulum made from pure copper for finding suitable vegetables for a certain diet? (Answer: "yes" or "no.")

It is generally known that copper is an excellent conductor and will pass on any form of energy very well. But while copper has a purifying effect, it is nevertheless in its natural form very poisonous! It reacts strongly to all kinds of natural energies and quickly becomes oxygen. You can test this with a simple experiment: place a thin piece of red copper (for example, a penny) in fresh tomato juice and wait for some time —the result of this experiment is surprising! At first, the copper shines quite beautifully, then it will gradually dissolve, although this process might take a long time.

In this particular case, it would not be a good idea to use a pendulum made of copper, as the strong reactions of this metal might stand in the way of an objective answer to health issues.

The Thread or the Chain on the Pendulum

An indispensable accessory is, of course, the thread or the chain on which the pendulum hangs. It can be a thread made from a natural material, such as, for example, silk, flax, or some other—preferably finely spun—fabric. It can also be a silver chain that is made from round chain links, if possible, so that the energy is passed on as equally as possible. There are no firm rules for the thread or the chain; some people prefer natural materials, and to others it does not matter.

The length of the thread or the chain on the pendulum should be regulated so that the pendulum can move unhindered; however, it should not be too long; if so, your emotional contact with the pendulum could be lost. If you don't hold the thread firmly, the passing on of information could get complicated; so coordinate the pendulum and the length of the thread very carefully. After you have experimented with different pendulums and different lengths of thread regarding material, shape, and size, you will notice that one thread or chain fits to each material, to each size, or to each shape of the pendulum, and is "exactly right."

Some Guidelines for Selecting the Pendulum

While a pendulum can be made from any kind of material, there is one final consideration to take into account: the purpose for which the pendulum is going to be used. If you are going to question physical problems, eating habits, or precious stones, for example, don't use a heavy brass pendulum. If the questions you will be asking are more theoretical, you can use any type. Pay attention to the fact, though, that a pendulum of precious stone or metal should fit your own character and supplement possible emotional deficits. Someone with a melancholy character, for example, could be put out completely if he worked with a pendulum made from dark obsidian or steel; rock crystal, aquamarine, or silver would be a better choice for him.

In short, the usefulness of the pendulum will show up in practice! Because of this, try out a variety of pendulums to see what shapes and materials suit you best and are most effective. You will want to work with several pendulums in different situations or with different questions.

If you find the right pendulum at last, it will be, thanks to its composition, its weight, its shape, and its mobility, a very sensitive measuring instrument for the picking up of energy or radiations. You can then also use it as an aid in expanding of your possibilities, complementing your knowledge, and helping you to better understand yourself and your fellow humans.

The Movement of the Pendulum

The most important feature of a weight on a piece of thread or on a chain is, as already mentioned, its movement towards one spot—where the force of attraction of the earth is greatest. Energy sets the pendulum in motion, and if this energy falls away, the pendulum eventually comes to a standstill. Once again, each life form has its own individual energy (oscillation), as it is surrounded by its individual aura of cosmic radiation. We can pick up this radiation with the very sensitive pendulum, and when we do, it will begin to oscillate.

The pendulum does not oscillate arbitrarily; there are many specific pendulum figures. It can move, for example, from left to right (horizontal oscillations), from top to bottom (vertical oscillations) or make circular movements either to the right or to the left side.

What meaning this oscillation has (pendulum swing) and how we can interpret it will be the topic of the following chapter (see the section: The Determination of the Individual Code).

Preparing for Work with the Pendulum

Can anyone make the pendulum oscillate?

Yes, in principle, anyone can use the pendulum; there is no "educational training" necessary to be a diviner. However, some practice and experience are recommended so that the information the pendulum offers can be interpreted faithfully. The matter with which the pendulum works is very subtle, and the pendulum is a very sensitive instrument.

Practice and experience are there for the asking if you work with the pendulum on a regular basis. First of all, you need to become acquainted with one or even several pendulums, and determine your individual pendulum code, in order to get a feel for the different materials and their various radiations.

You will find exercises in the sections entitled What does a pendulum look like?, Determining your individual code, and Getting in touch. Do not, under any circumstances, skip these exercises. If you practice things in the right way and on a regular basis, and then compare the resulting oscillations with one another, you'll get sufficient experience with that alone!

Personal preparation

What precisely is included in "preparation time"? First and foremost, it is very important that you get ready mentally for work with the pendulum. This holds true not only for the practical, hands-on aspects, but also for the environment, for the matter you wish to work with, in dealing with disturbances, and so on. In short, everything that could be of importance plays a role in personal preparation.

For this reason, it's wise to create an optimal work situation. If your surroundings permit you to get distracted easily, and if you have the extra space, it might make sense to set up a special room for working with the pendulum (see section: Setting up a Pendulum Room).

Good preparation means that the pendulum results will not be influenced in a negative way. The more that psychological and physical disturbances are excluded, the more precise will be your results.

Am I willing to be open and honest?

When you prepare yourself for work with the pendulum, you need to focus on it exclusively, and remain undistracted by any kind of irrelevant thought or circumstances. This preparation means getting mentally prepared for what can happen and posing the questions: "Am I willing to be honest towards the information I might receive? Am I in a position to remain neutral towards what can possibly take place?"

The following guidelines will help you with your mental preparation:

- Get in touch with your subconscious by concentrating on your personal "I." Close your eyes and breathe calmly in and out for about a minute. If your respiration is still calm after this period of time, remain still and breathe calmly for another minute. You will have established contact when you feel warmth flowing through your body.

- Put your mind into neutral and release all thoughts that are linked with the pendulum work; in this way, you will be more receptive.

- Open up—both for possible diverse questions as well as for information that can be quite varied and sometimes even surprise you greatly.

- Be neutral towards the possible results and try to relax as much as possible. Be entirely aware of the fact that you are "only" a mediator between the radiation and energies around you and the pendulum in your hand.

- Be willing to receive any kind of cosmic or human "wavelength." Apart from your unconscious, you must also get in touch with the materials or persons you wish to work with. This requires some practice! (See section: Getting in touch).

- Be entirely honest and do not let yourself be distracted by any kind of compelling motives of your own or others, to achieve a particular result. It may even come about that the pendulum will not give any answer, or that the answer will not be enough if the moment or circumstances are not (yet) ripe!

- Don't give up too quickly, as many disturbing factors can play a role; you will first have to look for them before you can exclude them. For example, the position in which you are working may be incorrect, or you may be greatly distracted by objects or influences in your immediate surroundings. Perhaps you have not asked the question correctly. Eliminate these disturbing factors as much as possible and try again.

How do I need to hold the pendulum?

Hold the pendulum so that it can move unhindered. The thread must be long enough for it to swing. Especially in the beginning, it is relatively difficult to handle the pendulum correctly without influencing its movement physically. You may be holding the pendulum incorrectly so that it cannot move freely, or perhaps you have not yet found the correct position through which the pendulum gets a "thrust." In order to be certain that you are holding it correctly, here are a few examples of the correct positioning of the pendulum.

Position 1

Use a pendulum that has a thread or chain long enough to be adjusted easily at will.

- Wind the end of the thread or the chain around your little finger so that the thread does not hang down loosely (which can be distracting).
- Hold the thread or the chain in a relaxed way but firmly between your thumb and index finger, letting the pendulum hang loosely.
- Now turn the palm of your hand upward and let the thread, on which the pendulum hangs, easily glide between your thumb and index finger.
- Do not try to prop up your arm on the table (especially in the beginning, this can be quite difficult), as you will leave too little "freedom" for the pendulum.
- Push your elbow slightly against your body, so that your lower arm is able to rest: in this way, your body position is both relaxed and receptive.

Position 2

- Follow the first three steps of position 1; here, however, your palm points downward.
- Relax your entire hand, but have enough strength to keep a firm hold on the pendulum.

- If you have not yet had a lot of experience, rest your arm lightly on the table; try, however, not to bend back your wrist.
- Your thumb and lower arm make a straight line: in this way, your position is both relaxed and receptive.

Position 3

There is another position of the hand that is sometimes used, in which the pendulum is held by one finger only:

- Use a thread or chain that is long enough that its length can be regulated.
- Make a relaxed fist and stretch your index finger forward as if you're pointing at something.
- Wind the thread once or twice around your index finger and let the pendulum hang down loosely. The length of the thread or the chain must, of course, be sufficient to allow for this.
- Wind the end of the thread or the chain around your little finger; be sure that you have enough "elbow room" so that the pendulum is not influenced.
- Now press your elbow slightly against your body and turn the palm of your hand upward so that you can see your fingers.
- Or slightly prop up your elbow on the table. Turn your palm downward (you will see the knuckles of your fingers) and make a straight line with your index finger and lower arm. Be sure you don't bend back your wrist.

With which hand should I set the pendulum in motion? People have different opinions. Some claim that it's best to set the pendulum in motion with the hand you write with; others claim that you should use the other hand. The hand you write with supposedly symbolizes rational thinking; the other hand mirrors your emotional, intuitive, and unconscious side. Others claim exactly the opposite, that the hand you write with mirrors the emotional, intuitive, and unconscious. In practice, people often find out right away which hand is better to make the pendulum oscillate. And with practice and experience, the diviner will come to feel which hand "conducts" better. It is even possible that this will change after a time—or change back; there are no irrefutable rules.

If you are, after the previous exercises and explanations, holding the pendulum correctly without tension or fatigue, and you are able to feel which hand is your "pendulum hand," then the moment has come in which to establish your individual code.

It is easy to establish it with the exercises below. Even if you have a lot of experience, it's a good idea to check this code every once in a while in order to limit as much as possible any uncertainty regarding your results.

Determining one's individual code

The individual code of the oscillation of the pendulum is so named because it varies for every individual. If you want to work with the pendulum, it is essential to first determine your own pendulum code, valid only for you, in order to be able to make the pendulum oscillate infallibly.

The individual code is connected with different, firmly established figures that the pendulum describes. With the help of the exercises below, you will determine very quickly which designs appear most in your work, what they mean, and how to assess them.

To determine your pendulum code you first need to establish contact with your unconscious. Working with the pendulum means basically making visible the information that lies in your unconscious.

How do you proceed?

Take a large piece of paper or thin cardboard, preferably a white one, and place it on a flat surface—on a table, for example. Take the pendulum in your hand (in the correct pendulum position) and hold it completely still over a certain spot on the paper. Relax and set your spirit free of superfluous thoughts. Focus your eyes on the pendulum. After some time you will be able to "feel" the pendulum: it will seem heavier and swing in a certain direction. Now you are in touch with your pendulum.

As you will always have a question when working with the pendulum, it is necessary to find out which motion signals a positive result ("yes") and which one a negative result ("no").

Pose a question to the pendulum, the answer to which you know for certain—in this case "yes"—and observe the movement the pendulum makes.

Pose another question. Watch which motion appears most often for "yes," or which one is the strongest. If you don't succeed right then, or if the motion of the pendulum is not very obvious, repeat the exercise after a short break. If you are distracted or cannot concentrate, figure out what disturbing factors might be playing a role. Eliminate them and repeat the exercise.

If you succeed in achieving a clear movement after a few attempts, draw this movement with a pencil on a sheet of paper or piece of cardboard. It does not necessarily have to be one single line: let your hand follow the movement several times and thoroughly observe the result. Clearly assign importance to this indicated movement—in this case "yes"—and write this in big letters on the sheet of paper or on the piece of cardboard. Now you will know for sure which movement means "yes."

After this exercise, try to have the pendulum make an opposing motion—in this case with the meaning "no"—by posing a question to which the answer will be a hundred percent "no." Observe the oscillations of the pendulum, draw them on a sheet of paper and write the meaning next to it.

If the pendulum, in this exercise, happens to swing in a circular movement you might interpret that as meaning something entirely different—for example, "perhaps," or "the question is still unclear," or "this question cannot or must not be answered at this time." Draw these movements on the sheet of paper as well and write the meaning next to them.

Once you have done the above-mentioned exercises often enough that you have no doubts about the meaning of the oscillations, do the exercises with your eyes closed. Relax and put your mind into neutral. Let the pendulum hang entirely motionless before you concentrate on the motions the pendulum is supposed to carry out. If you know for sure that the pendulum is moving, open your eyes in order to copy the movement on the sheet of paper. Write down once again whether the meaning is in agreement with the movement you perceived with closed eyes.

Only when can you carry out this last exercise successfully can you be sure that you have the "feel" of the pendulum really under control.

Note that the motions of the pendulum might also be influenced by the "oscillated object" itself, by your working method, or by your lack of experience as the diviner. So, carry out

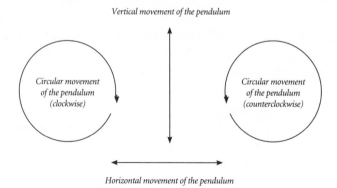

Vertical movement of the pendulum

Circular movement
of the pendulum
(clockwise)

Circular movement
of the pendulum
(counterclockwise)

Horizontal movement of the pendulum

these exercises with a series of pendulums (different sizes, shapes, materials, weights, etc.) and determine how the movements of the pendulum are influenced by these variations.

Start a collection of the drawings so that all the possible motions of the pendulum become familiar to you and potential misunderstandings can be eliminated. Practice and experiment with these drawings for some time before really working with the pendulum. It is not important whether the pendulum makes great or small movements; concentrate exclusively on the direction of the oscillation.

Establishing contact

"Contact" is an essential part of the work with the pendulum. In the previous section we saw that we have to establish contact with both the pendulum and our unconscious before determining our individual code; it is, however, important for reliable pendulum results that we establish contact with the "oscillated object" as well.

It is relatively simple to establish contact with the pendulum. If you focus on the pendulum as it hangs down motionless, you will feel after some time that it is getting heavier and heavier and then seems to swing in a certain direction. Not everyone has the same experience; some experience it as a tickling or prickling, while others feel only the "heaviness."

If you want to figure out whether a pendulum or some other object is suitable to use in a particular situation, it is essential to make contact with it. If it is lying on the table in front of you, take it in your hand or touch it lightly. Concentrate on it and, if necessary, close your eyes. Let the aura of cosmic radiation have its effect upon you; feel the energy the object radiates. If this energy feels like a regular rhythm, you have established contact and you will feel the "wavelength" of the object clearly. Take your time in establishing this contact. It is especially important to have good contact with the object when you are searching for possible causes of aches and pains or illnesses. Establish contact by observing it or touching it, and then let the radiation sink in. Go ahead and close your eyes, although this is not absolutely necessary. What is of the greatest importance is your concentration and why you wish to establish this contact.

If you feel that the "cosmic" contact is at its optimal level, determine the "wavelength" in your mind. You may have to fall back on it at any time, especially if you have several questions in regard to one person. Also, include the personal aura of this person in this "elementary sketch." Should you feel a strong contrast between these two "sketches," it could be meaningful to learn, with all due caution, a little more about it—for example, with the help of the pendulum.

In the event that the object is not at your disposal, concentrate instead on a picture—a photo or detailed description—of the object or a thing that replaces the object. Such an object could be, for example, something that belonged to the person who paid particular attention to it, or for whom it was worth a great deal. If this is not the case, the remaining aura of the object will be too weak for oscillation.

Don't forget that every time you start over, you need to begin from a neutral, objective condition so that you can adapt to different wavelengths. Likewise, put your mind in neutral between various contacts and take a short break, if necessary.

You may also want to quickly wash your hands or get some fresh air so that you can set yourself free from the energy collected.

What kind of questions may I ask the pendulum?

You may ask the pendulum many kinds of questions on any number of topics, but it's important to take some basic rules into consideration. Whether or not your question can be answered depends on how you formulate your inquiry. For this reason, observe the following rules:

Basic rules

- Make your question as clear as possible: simple, short, and direct. Avoid sentences like: "Could it perhaps be possible that this decision might help me?" but rather ask: "Will this decision help me?"
- Do not pose two questions in one sentence, such as, for example: "Will it be sunny or cloudy tomorrow?"
- Always pose the question positively, such as, for example "Is this (this decision) good?" Instead of "Is this decision bad?"
- Never ask for answers that you already know, unless you're still practicing and trying to determine your individual code.
- Pose questions only out of genuine interest, never merely out of curiosity.
- Never ask for answers with which you could (intentionally or accidentally) hurt others or bring some disadvantage to them.
- Never ask for the "Why," but pose the question in such a way that the answer ("yes" or "no," or one of the other answers from the pendulum chart) will show you the way. Never ask for the result of bets or gambling.
- Be aware of the fact that it is difficult to make the pendulum oscillate for yourself, as it is seldom possible to obtain the necessary distance from your own self.

Therefore, pay attention to formulating your question correctly. If you do not follow these basic rules, you will not receive a reliable answer. If, for example, several different factors play a role, your question will be too complex to be answered all at once. Also, if the intention behind your query will not allow for the correct working of the pendulum, an unreliable answer will result.

The following questions or formulations should therefore be avoided:

Wrong questions or formulations

- Complicated, combined questions such as: "Do I have to take my jacket or my umbrella with me in case it is going to rain later on?"
- Questions posed out of negative emotions or intentions such as jealousy, rage, etc.
- Questions that come down to an involuntary "wrangling out" of information (out of curiosity).
- Unclear questions or questions that lend themselves to several interpretations.
- Questions to which the answers are already known in advance.
- Questions that hurt others or could bring harm to others, for example: "Has the nice person X the predisposition to get the terrible disease Y?"

There are no firm rules as to what topic the pendulum may be asked about; it depends very much upon how you formulate the question and with what kind of intention. You may, for example, ask questions regarding personal matters, find out about hitherto unknown causes of a lingering illness, or simply make the right choice from a variety of possibilities.

The following areas offer sufficient possibilities for pendulum work:

Suitable areas and topics with which you can work

- Reasons for suffering or illnesses
- Blockages of chakras and meridians
- Persons and relations to others, talents, characteristics, etc.
- Plants, minerals, etc. For example, "Does this person/this precious stone/this plant or this alternative medical treatment work for me?"
- Right nutrition or right eating habits

- Professional orientation (what are my ambitions or talents?)
- Application of alternative remedies (in this case, always consult your doctor or medical practitioner as well)
- Self-awareness (social behavior, talents, etc.)
- Relations to others (private or professional)
- Connections with other esoteric areas (such as astrology and Tarot)
- Environment (what has a good or negative influence on me?)

There are, of course, also areas that are not or are barely suitable for work with the pendulum. These are areas whose roots lie in a specific esoteric technique that is based on, for example, calculation, a traditional system, a particular (esoteric) technique or a traditional theory. Examples of these include:

- Astrology
- Aura reading, etc.
- Ayurveda
- I-Ching
- Reiki
- Tarot

Nevertheless, this book contains pendulum charts for several areas that are usually considered less suitable for oscillating. They were included in order to show that the starting point can still be decisive for the further suitability of a certain topic or area. If, for example, specific information about astrological data is missing, it is quite possible to supplement it with the help of the pendulum.

This can also happen if, for example, you're using a combined approach, based on intuition or "unconscious preference." An example here is the drawing of a Tarot card when laying out the cards. Therefore, some pendulum charts regarding this topic are also given in this book.

Disturbing factors when working with the pendulum

Another very important—in fact, indispensable—way of preparing for work with the pendulum is to take into consideration the circumstances and surroundings in which the pendulum has to function. Examine the nature and influences of any potentially disturbing factors and take measures to limit them as much as possible.

For the oscillation itself, good conductivity is the most important precondition. This means that not only the material of the pendulum, but also the place at which one works with the pendulum, has to have good conductivity and let through all the radiation that surrounds us.

If a lot of insulating material was used when the room in which you're working was set up, it is possible that could influence the results in a negative way. If, however, mainly natural building materials, which conduct energy well, were used, it will not influence the result.

This also holds true for the desk on which we work and the chair on which we sit. Wooden tables and chairs are very good conductors; the tabletop and seating should be made from natural materials. Before working with the pendulum, remove all metallic objects from your desk and be sure to avoid synthetics, such as plastic, for example, in your immediate surrounding. Remove all superfluous objects from your desk; place on it only those things with which you wish to work, such as the pendulum chart, the object to be oscillated and, if you want, your favorite tablecloth (you may, of course, also work at an "unset" table).

Also, your posture is important; generally, sit straight at the table at which you wish to work, feet flat on the ground next to each other at a distance of about four inches (10cm) apart, with toes pointing forward. In this way, you are not only well "grounded," but you can also remain in this stable, relaxed position for some time.

By all means possible, you will need to focus your attention one hundred percent in order to be able to concentrate properly on the pendulum! Be aware of where you leave your "free" hand (the hand that isn't holding the pendulum). Let this hand rest on the table or in your lap–palm up–so that it doesn't affect the movement of the pendulum. This hand position will also keep you from moving around any objects on the table, as this can be a disturbing factor.

Some people are sold on the idea of placing their free hand on their back in order to keep it out of play. But any position is fine as long as you don't think about what to do with your hand or where to keep it.

Also pay attention to the jewelry you might be wearing since it will be in the immediate reach of the pendulum as well! Better yet, don't wear any jewelry (not even a watch) when working with the pendulum.

Don't wear any clothes made from chemical fibers as they may influence the oscillation of the pendulum through their effect on the electromagnetic field as well as the "cosmic" radiation surrounding you.

In regard to shoes, their soles in particular can have a strong isolating effect on the radiation that surrounding you. If you notice that the pendulum is reacting badly or insufficiently, it might perhaps help if you take off your shoes; the difference should be noticeable immediately.

Switch off any apparatus that sends out electromagnetic radiation, such as your computer or television set; the standby switch of the equipment should be turned off as well, in order to avoid as much radiation as you possibly can.

If you wish to shield yourself from all kinds of disturbing factors, you may even insulate the legs of your table and chairs by placing them on glass, and insulate the surface of the tabletop with a glass cover, elastic, or linoleum. In this way, the pendulum chart, the material, or the pendulum itself is insulated optimally against magnetic radiation coming from the earth.

If it inspires you, you may want to listen to music at a low volume. But if you're just beginning to work with the pendulum, music will distract you rather than foster concentration.

Avoid smoking cigarettes during the time you are working with the pendulum as well as consuming alcohol or other stimulants that can influence your mood. If you are not completely sober and your mind is not entirely neutral, the results of your work will be influenced and the picture "clouded" so that the movements of the pendulum are no longer objective and become essentially unusable.

Sometimes it happens that, although you prepare as much as possible and have therefore eliminated all conceivable sources of interference, you notice that the oscillation of the pendulum does not "feel" good or is influenced by an unknown factor. Don't pay attention to any of the results received under these circumstances. Try again later on when these disturbances are often no longer active. It is also possible that you may not be using a suitable pendulum. Take another pendulum and start again.

In short, when working with the pendulum we have to take into consideration all the different kinds of sources of interference that can influence the result of the pendulum:

- Sources of interference from the pendulum: material, conductivity, etc.
- Sources of interference from the environment: insulating material, surrounding objects, etc.
- Sources of interference from the pendulum object: material, interaction with the pendulum, etc.
- Sources of interference in yourself: lack of experience, lack of contact with the pendulum or the object of the pendulum, false intentions, etc.

Setting Up a
Pendulum Room

Setting up your very own pendulum corner

As mentioned before, if you are working regularly with the pendulum or wish to work with it, it can be very pleasant to have a room that is specially set up for this purpose. The room does not need to be large; a "corner" is sufficient. Here you can create the atmosphere that feels just right to you. You may set up this "pendulum corner," for example, in the most pleasant or quietest room of your home.

Furnish this room with a (preferably) wooden table with at least two chairs. If possible, use natural materials and avoid electronic apparatus in your immediate surroundings. If you find it pleasant, you might place an evergreen plant close to you. Keep the room free of synthetics as much as possible. Place, for instance, mats made from rushes or a wool rug on the floor. Avoid as well sun protection made from synthetics or metal in your immediate surroundings, since these can act like a "shield."

What can you store here?

In this corner, furnished according to your own taste, you may also create special storage possibilities for your pendulums and other materials with which you are working, as well as for pendulum charts and insulating material. In this way, you will have stored them securely and they will not be exposed to any kind of neglect (dust, excessive sunlight, etc.) For example, you can set up a small cupboard in which you can keep both books on the topic as well as some smaller objects. In here, you may also store your pendulum equipment, your pendulum diary or your pendulum logbook (see next section). In essence, what you are doing is creating a corner with the right atmosphere and the right equipment, in which nothing prevents you from getting the best results possible.

The personal pendulum equipment

Immediately after your first attempts with the pendulum, you may assemble your personal pendulum equipment. For this purpose use a (wooden) box or case that is large enough to hold small utensils or materials. The size and shape of a sewing box or something like that is sufficient. In this box you can store all kinds of materials that you might need when working with the pendulum:

- Diverse pendulums (separated in bags)
- Diverse threads (cotton, flax, wool, etc.)
- Small pliers
- Diverse chains and links of chain (silver, gold, etc.)
- Cotton tissue (minimum 12 x 12 inches or 30 x 30cm) for the cleaning of pendulums made from brass and precious metal
- Small bottle with pure* water for cleaning pendulums made from crystal and precious stones.
  (*purified from negative influences and positively influenced by (visual) meditation, oscillation, etc.)
- You may also keep a notebook along with your other equipment in which you write down the results of your work with the pendulum. You may expand this "logbook" into a more detailed "pendulum diary" by adding drawings of your individual pendulum code, personal pendulum charts, and personal experiences and interpretations.

This can be very useful, as your personal experience may differ from the information in pendulum literature, such as this book. If you keep your diary faithfully, it will develop into your personal pendulum workbook.

Storage, cleaning, and loading
of the pendulum

Any object you use often or intensively should be cleaned regularly. There are different ways of doing this—which one you use depends on the material of the pendulum and the intensity of your work. Here, we make a distinction between pendulums made from crystal and precious stone and those made from precious metal or alloy.

Pendulums made from crystal or precious stone

Pendulums made from a natural or porous material need careful treatment.

Therefore, don't use tap water or—even more harmful—salt water for the cleaning of the pendulum since it can contain substances that may seep into the stone or the crystal. This can not only alter the "cosmic" aura, but it may also damage your pendulum irreparably! The effect of salt may, for example, be that your pendulum breaks apart after some time. Furthermore, your pendulum may take on an unpleasant color, so that you'll have to search for a new pendulum if you are working with colors.

Generally only use clean or distilled water that is purified from all negative "cosmic influences." You may purify the water yourself without any great difficulty through (visual) meditation, oscillation (with a new pendulum from brass or copper), or by gripping the bottle with both hands for about a minute.

Rinse the pendulum carefully and place it in a dark area for drying. Do not leave it in the sun as the rays can alter it permanently or even damage it. Never place a spherically cut or molded pendulum made from lead-crystal in the sun as it can have the same effect as a magnifying glass and could cause a fire!

Cut or polished pendulums are slightly less sensitive, as they are often less porous. Yet the same precautions hold true: prefer safe things to unsafe things and treat your pendulum with respect and care.

When your pendulum has been cleaned thoroughly and has rested for 24 hours, it is once again loaded and ready for use. If your pendulum is very "exhausted," you may also let it rest for more than a day; one week should be enough in most instances. Don't let pendulums made from other natural, porous material such as wood, get wet. Water or dampness might harm the natural structure, resulting in the pendulum being less suitable for its work. Never place pendulums of such natural material in the sun; excessive sunlight or too much warmth may harm them as well. Cleanse these sensitive pendulums as little as possible. When they must be cleansed, the best method is to grip the pendulum with both hands, so that the negative energy may flow away through your body. Let the pendulum rest for about two days after the cleansing and then use it only for "subtle" questions for a while.

Pendulums from metal

Metal pendulums can withstand a lot, but do not use water to cleanse them! In some cases, water can even oxidize the pendulum. As this kind of pendulum is barely or not at all porous, it is sufficient to rub it well with a piece of cotton; this will remove most of the pollution caused by disturbances of "cosmic energy" through interfering radiation, such as electromagnetic radiation or other very strong energies.

If the "cosmic energy" of the pendulum is strongly disturbed, you can cleanse it with a pendulum made from crystal or precious stone. Place the polluted pendulum on your desk and hold the pendulum made from crystal or precious stone above it for about 10 minutes. The disturbed energy is thus neutralized, and the pendulum can be used again immediately afterwards. Pendulums made from precious metal or alloys do not need to rest for 24 hours!

Also try not to place pendulums in the sun or in another warm spot (close to a radiator, for example). Don't keep them close to an electromagnetic source of energy or any other type of strong radiation. Avoid those "hidden magnets" that are, for instance, contained in audio apparatus.

For safety reasons, keep your pendulums in a container made from wood or glass, which will protect them against most harmful radiation. Do not store pendulums from various metals or from alloys together in the same container. Instead, try to keep them separated, for instance, in a container made of wood or in a bag made of cotton or silk. In this way you can prevent the pendulums, especially if they are not used very often, from influencing each other. This will also protect them against small damage such as scratches.

Preparation for Work with Pendulum Charts

Before you start working with the pendulum charts, a few hints might be useful about how to use them.

How is the pendulum chart put together?

Choose from 15 or 25 possibilities

In this book, you will find two types of pendulum charts—ones with 15 possible answers and ones with 25 possible answers. Actually, any number of answers would be acceptable, but individuals are not always able to work equally well with different numbers. In this book 15 and 25 circular segments were chosen. It would be very difficult to work well with any more than 25 answers on one pendulum chart.

Order of possible answers

The order of the answers on circular pendulum charts runs counterclockwise. This, however, exists solely as a piece of information; in itself, it has no influence on the work with the pendulum, but just explains where the order of answers begins and where it stops. This makes it a little easier to use the chart, because in some cases, explanations of the answers do not fit on the chart itself and you will find them with their corresponding numbers on the left-hand page. This does not influence the pendulum either, since the pendulum looks for its path all by itself. Since the chart is circular, it does not need to lie in a certain position. It doesn't matter whether it stands right-side-up or upside-down.

One question, two answers

Usually two charts are assigned to questions about one particular topic. One pendulum chart answers the question in a positive manner ("does this work for me?") and the other chart answers the question in a negative way ("Should I avoid this?"). This concept was used in order to eliminate certain faulty conclusions. If no clear answer is given with the pendulum, then this could mean either that no answer is possible or that all answers should be excluded! Both could be wrong. It is certainly conceivable that one clear answer might be impossible, but you can't establish whether or not one of the possible answers should be disregarded. This does not help the questioner very much, as the answer you're getting tells little about the situation itself. In order to explain this situation in greater detail, the second chart was created, which tackles the question from a different angle; it should deliver the additional information you want.

Possible answer "not on this chart"

Each pendulum chart contains the possible answer "not on this chart." This means that either several (unknown) answers will fit the question posed or that one single answer is not possible; in this case, though, it indicates that the question is not relevant. However, you can question the following chart in regard to the same topic or, as a last possibility, you yourself can create an additional and supplemental chart for this topic.

Indirect question—indirect answer

It is also possible that the pendulum will give an indirect answer to a question that has not been posed (yet). If remedies are being selected—such as medicinal herbs, ethereal oils, etc.—a subliminal illness might be discovered for which no question has been posed up to this point. Take this answer seriously and come back to it at a later time.

Suffering and remedies

With all remedies, you will find the note that you should consult your doctor or medical practitioner for the right application of medicinal herbs. This precautionary measure should not be disregarded. Though the pendulum may be a good adviser, it is not a doctor . . .

Recommendations for further reading

Some pendulum charts contain recommendations for further readings on the topic discussed; this is merely complementary material. It is often wise to read a little more on a complex topic, which can be more confusing in application than is easily processed in a pendulum chart (for example: colors and their application, etc.) In this way, you may be able to improve your knowledge and apply it later on when making the pendulum oscillate.

Explanatory note to the pendulum chart

On the left-hand page, you will find the row of possible answers repeated in the same order as in the chart, but often with additional details. The chart itself often lacks the space needed to get all the information in. On this page, in addition, you will sometimes find references to other pendulum charts. Always read this page carefully!

Creating an additional pendulum chart

In some cases it might turn out that the pendulum charts at hand contain too little information. You might, for example, have questioned all the charts on one topic and keep receiving the answer "not in this chart."

In these cases, an additional pendulum chart might be helpful. At the end of this book, you will find two "blank" pendulum charts for your use in creating your own charts. If you prefer more or fewer possible answers, you may certainly opt for another arrangement.

Draw a circle and divide it into the desired number of segments. Note, however, that you may be confused in regard to the possible answers if you've come up with an even number of segments. Working with a semicircle will eliminate that confusion.

Final Practical Preparations

You may achieve good results with your pendulum if you are distracted as little as possible. It also helps if you put these finishing touches on your preparation.

- Take your time setting out all objects you will need. If there are many, because you're using the pendulum for a number of different materials or want to use quite a lot of pendulum charts, don't place all of them on the table at which you're working. Have them handy, for example, on a stool or a side table placed beside your desk.
- Check on whether or not you have the right pendulum for the job, and decide, if necessary, on several pendulums. Once again, don't place all of them on the desk; choose one and place the others on the side table.
- Observe the pendulum charts or the objects to be questioned and then decide if you have chosen the right ones or if perhaps something is still missing. Are you missing a pendulum chart? Do you have all the materials that you wish to use?
- Now wash your hands thoroughly. Since you have touched so many different objects and encountered so many thoughts, you would do well to "cleanse" yourself carefully before concentrating on your work with the pendulum. Washing your hands is also an excellent way to allow negative energy, which might have accumulated in your body, to flow away. And using

natural materials that have conductive characteristics helps things along, since negative energy can flow away into the ground.

- Pick one pendulum and one pendulum chart, which you believe are most suitable at this moment, and place them on the table.
- Sit at the table and take the pendulum into your hand. Let your "free" hand rest on the table or in your lap (or on your back); above all else, you need to feel comfortable in your position.
- Breathe deeply and calmly a few times in order to expel thoughts that can distract you from your inner peace. Be receptive and decide to wait and see what results you get. You may be curious, but first and foremost you need to be neutral. Concentrate on the pendulum and establish contact with it.
- Be receptive to all kinds of information that may reach you through the pendulum. Realize that you are a "medium" between "cosmic" radiation, the energy that surrounds us, and the sensitive measuring instrument with which you are working.
- Concentrate on the question; your thoughts are positive.
- Now formulate your question briefly and precisely; try to avoid any vagueness and let the pendulum work . . .
- May the pendulum be an invaluable tool for you—for life!

Pendulum Charts

CHART I

When should I use the pendulum today?

1. now
2. in the morning
3. in the afternoon
4. in the evening
5. at night
6. the entire day
7. day and night
8. in half an hour
9. in one hour
10. at a later time today
11. after minor preparations
12. after intensive preparations
13. after work
14. during a break
15. not on this chart

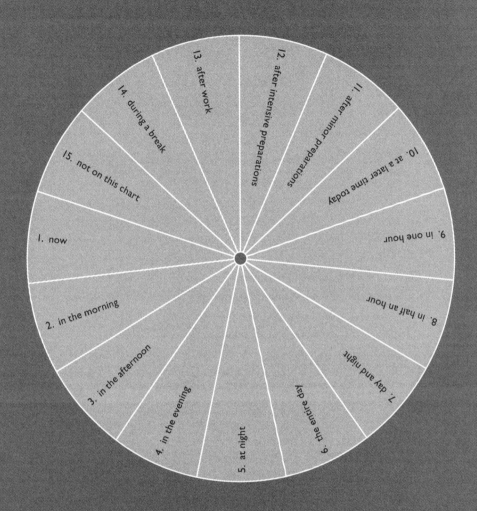

1. now
2. in the morning
3. in the afternoon
4. in the evening
5. at night
6. the entire day
7. day and night
8. in half an hour
9. in one hour
10. at a later time today
11. after minor preparations
12. after intensive preparations
13. after work
14. during a break
15. not on this chart

When should I use the pendulum today?

CHART 2

How reliable is my intuition—at this moment?

1. not or hardly at all
2. 0–15%
3. 15–25%
4. 25–50%
5. 50–65%
6. 65–75%
7. 75–85%
8. 85–95%
9. 95–99.9%
10. 99.9–100%
11. not measurable—environment
12. not measurable—personal factors
13. not measurable—outer influences
14. not measurable—personal influence
15. not on this chart

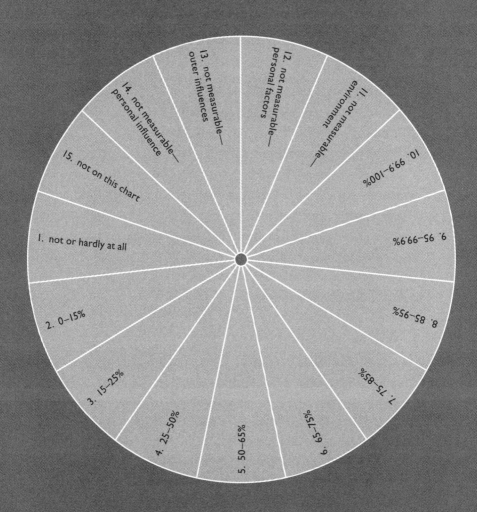

12. not measurable—
personal factors

11. not measurable—
environment

10. 99.9–100%

9. 95–99.9%

8. 85–95%

7. 75–85%

6. 65–75%

5. 50–65%

4. 25–50%

3. 15–25%

2. 0–15%

1. not or hardly at all

15. not on this chart

14. not measurable—
personal influence

13. not measurable—
outer influences

How reliable is my intuition—at this moment?

CHART 3

On what topic areas can I work the pendulum best today?

1. health—nutrition
2. health—body care and lifestyle habits
3. health—main topics (physical spiritual)
4. health—illnesses/suffering (physical)
5. health—(physical and spiritual)
6. health—remedies (internal)
7. health—remedies (internal, external)
8. inner growth and spirituality
9. inner growth and spirituality (helpers)
10. personal characteristics
11. education, profession, and talent
12. friendship and relationship
13. relaxation, sport, and fun
14. environmental factors
15. not on this chart

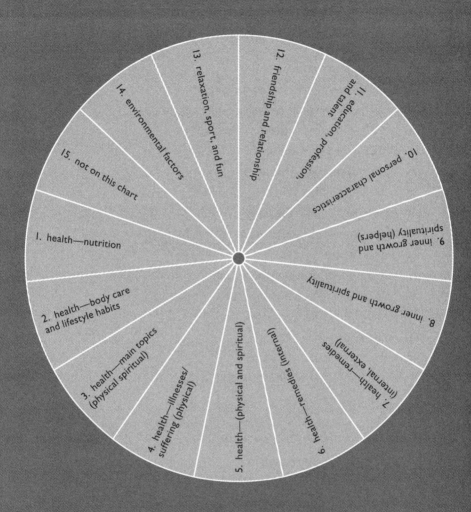

On what topic areas can I work the pendulum best today?

13. relaxation, sport, and fun

14. environmental factors

15. not on this chart

1. health—nutrition

2. health—body care and lifestyle habits

3. health—main topics (physical spiritual)

4. health—illnesses/ suffering (physical)

5. health—(physical and spiritual)

6. health—remedies (internal)

7. health—remedies (internal, external)

8. inner growth and spirituality

9. inner growth and spirituality (helpers)

10. personal characteristics

11. education, profession, and talent

12. friendship and relationship

CHART 4

What topic areas should I avoid today?

1. health—nutrition
2. health—body care and lifestyle habits
3. health—main topics (physical, spiritual)
4. health—illnesses/suffering (physical)
5. health—(physical and spiritual)
6. health—remedies (internal)
7. health—remedies (internal, external)
8. inner growth and spirituality
9. inner growth and spirituality (helpers)
10. personal characteristics
11. education, profession, and talent
12. friendship and relationship
13. relaxation, sport, and fun
14. environmental factors
15. not on this chart

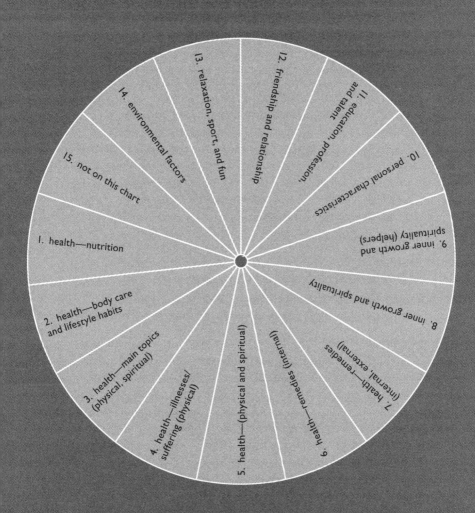

What topic areas should I avoid today?

CHART 5

Which chart contains the best information regarding my question?

1. health—nutrition: nutrients
2. health—nutrition: allergy
3. health—nutrition: taste and diet
4. health—body care and lifestyle habits
5. health—main topics
6. health—illnesses/suffering: localization
7. health—illnesses/suffering: condition
8. health—illnesses/suffering: allergies
9. health—illnesses/suffering: chakras
10. health—illnesses/suffering: meridians
11. health—illnesses: chakra/meridian
12. health—remedies: nutritional support
13. health—remedies: medicinal herbs
14. health—remedies: alternative medical
15. health—remedies: minerals, metals
16. health—remedies: colors
17. health—remedies: meditation
18. inner growth and spirituality
19. inner growth and spirituality: oracle
20. personal characteristics and abilities
21. education, profession, and talent
22. friendship and relationship
23. relaxation, sport, and fun
24. environment
25. not on this chart

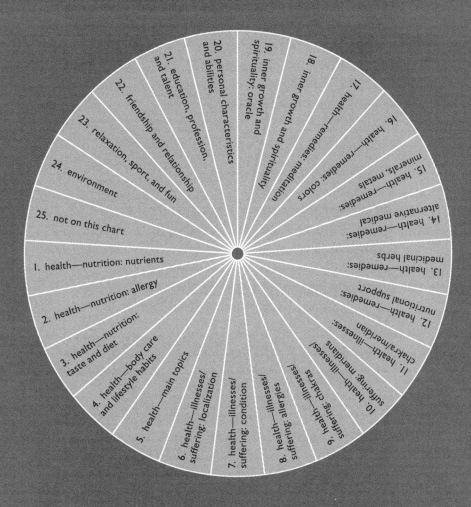

1. health—nutrition: nutrients
2. health—nutrition: allergy
3. health—nutrition: taste and diet
4. health—body care and lifestyle habits
5. health—main topics
6. health—illnesses/suffering: localization
7. health—illnesses/suffering: condition
8. health—illnesses/suffering: allergies
9. health—illnesses/suffering: chakras
10. health—illnesses/suffering: meridians
11. health—illnesses: chakra/meridian
12. health—remedies: nutritional support
13. health—remedies: medicinal herbs
14. health—remedies: alternative medical
15. health—remedies: minerals, metals
16. health—remedies: colors
17. health—remedies: meditation
18. inner growth and spirituality
19. inner growth and spirituality: oracle
20. personal characteristics and abilities
21. education, profession, and talent
22. friendship and relationship
23. relaxation, sport, and fun
24. environment
25. not on this chart

Which chart contains the best information regarding my question?

CHART 6

I usually eat too little _____.

1. greens
2. fruits
3. fibers
4. vitamins
5. minerals
6. trace elements
7. proteins
8. carbohydrates
9. enzymes
10. nutritional supplements
11. bases
12. acids
13. antioxidants
14. fats
15. not on the chart

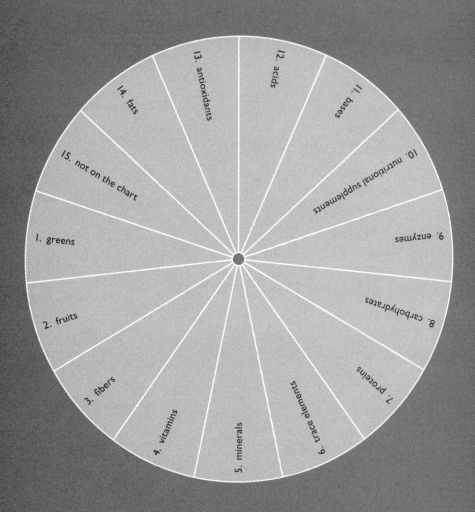

12. acids
11. bases
10. nutritional supplements
9. enzymes
8. carbohydrates
7. proteins
6. trace elements
5. minerals
4. vitamins
3. fibers
2. fruits
1. greens
15. not on the chart
14. fats
13. antioxidants

I usually eat too little _____.

CHART 7

I usually eat too much _____.

1. starch
2. sugar
3. fibers
4. vitamins
5. minerals
6. trace elements
7. proteins
8. carbohydrates
9. enzymes
10. nutritional supplements
11. bases
12. acids
13. antioxidants
14. fats
15. not on the chart

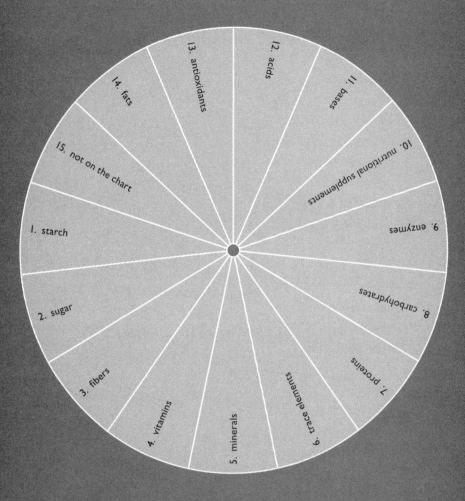

I usually eat too much _____.

CHART 8

What food do I eat too little of?

1. red fruits (berries)
2. citrus fruits
3. red meat
4. green vegetables
5. meats
6. freshwater fish
7. saltwater fish
8. crustaceans and shellfish
9. poultry
10. whole grains
11. red vegetables
12. milk and milk products
13. sour milk products
14. eggs
15. nuts, seeds, pips, etc.
16. potatoes, pumpkin, bananas, etc.
17. legumes
18. leafy vegetables
19. fruit vegetables
20. carrots, cabbage, tuber vegetables
21. spicy vegetables and hot spices
22. mushrooms
23. soy and soy products
24. whole grain rice and rice products
25. not on this chart

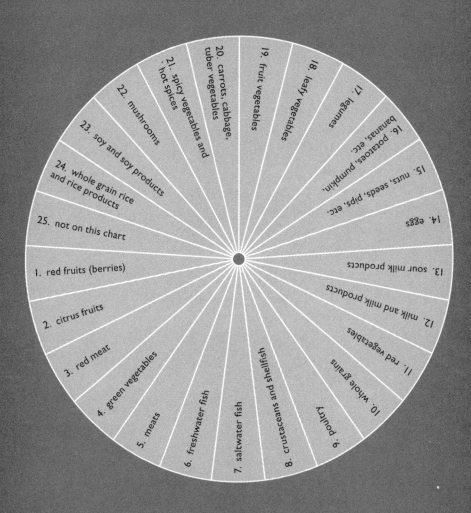

1. red fruits (berries)
2. citrus fruits
3. red meat
4. green vegetables
5. meats
6. freshwater fish
7. saltwater fish
8. crustaceans and shellfish
9. poultry
10. whole grains
11. red vegetables
12. milk and milk products
13. sour milk products
14. eggs
15. nuts, seeds, pips, etc.
16. potatoes, pumpkin, bananas, etc.
17. legumes
18. leafy vegetables
19. fruit vegetables
20. carrots, cabbage, tuber vegetables
21. spicy vegetables and hot spices
22. mushrooms
23. soy and soy products
24. whole grain rice and rice products
25. not on this chart

What food do I eat too little of?

CHART 9

What food should I be more moderate with?

1. red fruits (berries)
2. citrus fruits
3. red meat
4. green vegetables
5. meats
6. freshwater fish
7. saltwater fish
8. crustaceans and shellfish
9. poultry
10. whole grains
11. red vegetables
12. milk and milk products
13. sour milk products
14. eggs
15. nuts, seeds, pips, etc.
16. potatoes, pumpkin, bananas, etc.
17. legumes
18. leafy vegetables
19. fruit vegetables
20. carrots, cabbage, tuber vegetables
21. spicy vegetables and hot spices
22. mushrooms
23. soy and soy products
24. whole grain rice and rice products
25. not on this chart

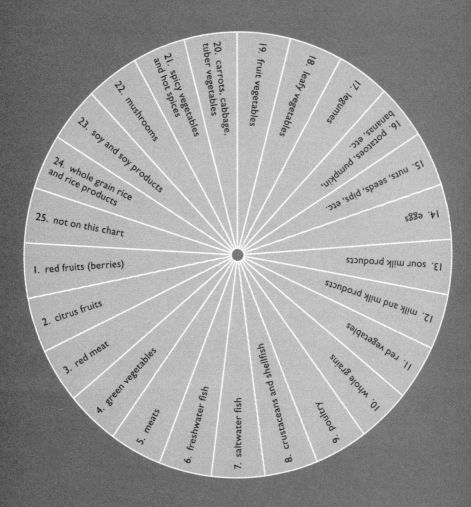

20. carrots, cabbage, tuber vegetables
21. spicy vegetables and hot spices
22. mushrooms
23. soy and soy products
24. whole grain rice and rice products
25. not on this chart
1. red fruits (berries)
2. citrus fruits
3. red meat
4. green vegetables
5. meats
6. freshwater fish
7. saltwater fish
8. crustaceans and shellfish
9. poultry
10. whole grains
11. red vegetables
12. milk and milk products
13. sour milk products
14. eggs
15. nuts, seeds, pips, etc.
16. potatoes, pumpkin, bananas, etc.
17. legumes
18. leafy vegetables
19. fruit vegetables

What food should I be more moderate with?

CHART 10

Which vitamins do I lack?

1. vitamin A (carotene)
2. vitamin B1 (thiamin)
3. vitamin B2 (riboflavin)
4. vitamin B3 (niacin)
5. vitamin B5 (pantothenic acid)
6. vitamin B6 (pyridoxine)
7. vitamin B9 (folic acid)
8. vitamin B12 (cyanocobalamin)
9. vitamin C (ascorbic acid)
10. vitamin D (ergosterol)
11. vitamin E (tocopherol)
12. vitamin F (essential fatty acids)
13. vitamin H (biotin)
14. vitamin K (coagulation vitamin)
15. vitamin P (rutin)

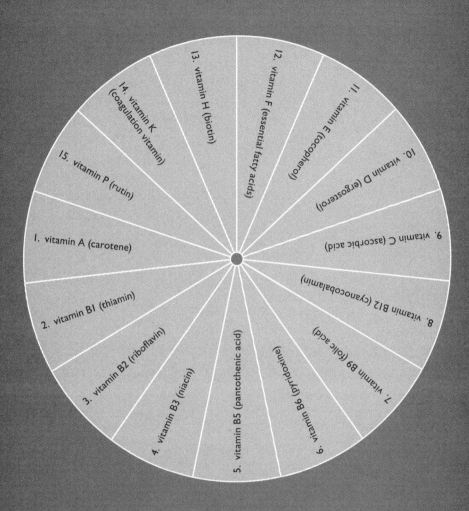

Which vitamins do I lack?

1. vitamin A (carotene)
2. vitamin B1 (thiamin)
3. vitamin B2 (riboflavin)
4. vitamin B3 (niacin)
5. vitamin B5 (pantothenic acid)
6. vitamin B6 (pyridoxine)
7. vitamin B9 (folic acid)
8. vitamin B12 (cyanocobalamin)
9. vitamin C (ascorbic acid)
10. vitamin D (ergosterol)
11. vitamin E (tocopherol)
12. vitamin F (essential fatty acids)
13. vitamin H (biotin)
14. vitamin K (coagulation vitamin)
15. vitamin P (rutin)

CHART II

Which minerals do I lack?

1. chromium
2. magnesium
3. calcium
4. potassium
5. sulfur
6. chlorine
7. fluorine
8. selenium
9. iron
10. zinc
11. copper
12. iodine
13. phosphorus
14. sodium
15. manganese

CONSULT YOUR DOCTOR BEFORE TAKING MINERALS!

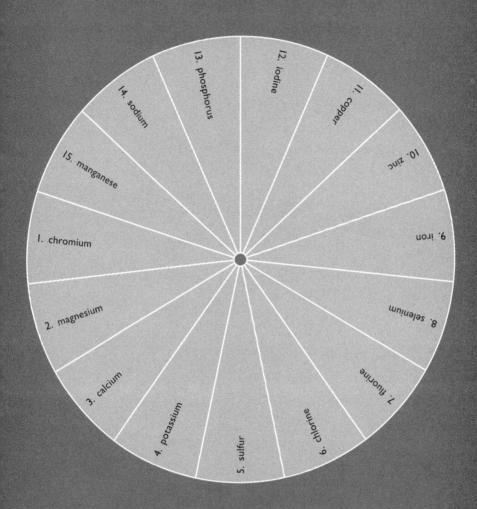

12. iodine
11. copper
10. zinc
9. iron
8. selenium
7. fluorine
6. chlorine
5. sulfur
4. potassium
3. calcium
2. magnesium
1. chromium
15. manganese
14. sodium
13. phosphorus

Which minerals do I lack?

CHART 12

What am I allergic to?

1. animal protein—meat
2. animal protein—fish
3. animal protein—poultry
4. animal protein—eggs
5. animal fats
6. diverse fats and oils
7. hot spices
8. odorous and flavoring substances
9. coloring substances
10. preservatives
11. wheat products with gluten
12. all kinds of wheat products
13. heavily digestive legumes
14. all legumes
15. crustaceans
16. shellfish
17. nuts, seeds, and pips
18. cow milk products
19. all milk products
20. refined sugar
21. various kinds of sugar
22. fermented products
23. strawberries
24. chocolate
25. not on this chart

SEE ALSO PENDULUM CHARTS 34, 35, 58, 117, 129.

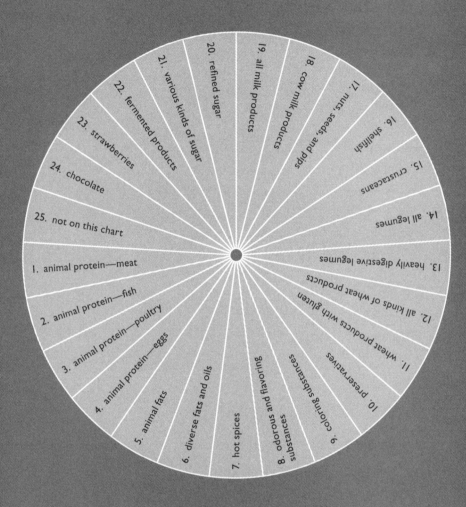

1. animal protein—meat
2. animal protein—fish
3. animal protein—poultry
4. animal protein—eggs
5. animal fats
6. diverse fats and oils
7. hot spices
8. odorous and flavoring substances
9. coloring substances
10. preservatives
11. wheat products with gluten
12. all kinds of wheat products
13. heavily digestive legumes
14. all legumes
15. crustaceans
16. shellfish
17. nuts, seeds, and pips
18. cow milk products
19. all milk products
20. refined sugar
21. various kinds of sugar
22. fermented products
23. strawberries
24. chocolate
25. not on this chart

What am I allergic to?

CHART 13

Which kind of taste suits me best?

1. sweet
2. sweet sour
3. sour
4. bitter
5. salty
6. spicy sweet
7. spicy salty
8. refreshingly sweet
9. refreshingly sour
10. fruity
11. fishy
12. well-seasoned
13. spicy
14. no special taste
15. not on this chart

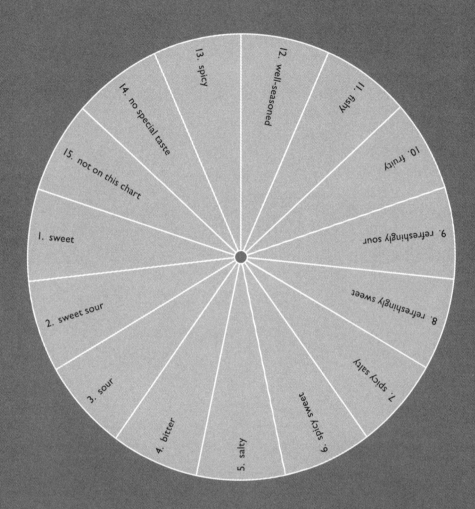

Which kind of taste suits me best?

CHART 14

Which kind of taste should I avoid?

1. sweet
2. sweet sour
3. sour
4. bitter
5. salty
6. spicy sweet
7. spicy salty
8. refreshingly sweet
9. refreshingly sour
10. fruity
11. fishy
12. well-seasoned
13. spicy
14. no special taste
15. not on this chart

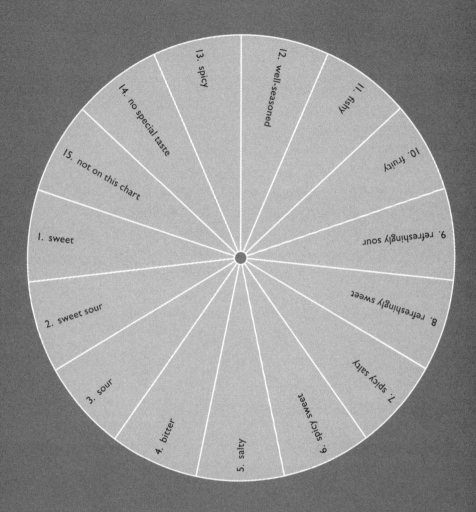

1. sweet
2. sweet sour
3. sour
4. bitter
5. salty
6. spicy sweet
7. spicy salty
8. refreshingly sweet
9. refreshingly sour
10. fruity
11. fishy
12. well-seasoned
13. spicy
14. no special taste
15. not on this chart

Which kind of taste should I avoid?

CHART 15

Which kind of diet (or nutrition) suits me best?

1. vegetarian food
2. lacto vegetable nutrition
3. vegan diet
4. ayurvedic diet
5. macrobiotic diet
6. fit for life diet
7. hypoglycemic diet
8. de-acidification therapy
9. Dr. Atkins diet
10. raw food diet
11. Pritikin diet
12. Hay diet
13. rotation diet
14. high protein diet
15. grapefruit diet
16. fasting
17. vegetable cure
18. less salt
19. less sugar
20. less fat
21. less meat
22. more fluids
23. (more) biologic nutrition/ products
24. more fresh vegetables and fruit
25. not on this chart

FASTING SHOULD BE CARRIED OUT ONLY UNDER THE SUPERVISION OF YOUR DOCTOR.

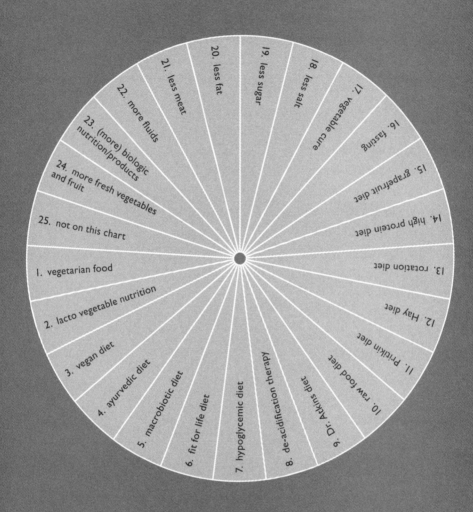

Which kind of diet (or nutrition) suits me best?

20. less fat
19. less sugar
21. less meat
18. less salt
22. more fluids
17. vegetable cure
23. (more) biologic nutrition/products
16. fasting
24. more fresh vegetables and fruit
15. grapefruit diet
25. not on this chart
14. high protein diet
1. vegetarian food
13. rotation diet
2. lacto vegetable nutrition
12. Hay diet
3. vegan diet
11. Pritikin diet
4. ayurvedic diet
10. raw food diet
5. macrobiotic diet
9. Dr. Atkins diet
6. fit for life diet
8. de-acidification therapy
7. hypoglycemic diet

CHART 16

Which kind of diet (or nutrition) should I avoid?

1. vegetarian food
2. lacto vegetable nutrition
3. vegan diet
4. ayurvedic diet
5. macrobiotic diet
6. fit for life diet
7. hypoglycemic diet
8. de-acidification therapy
9. Dr. Atkins diet
10. raw food diet
11. Pritikin diet
12. Hay diet
13. rotation diet
14. high protein diet
15. grapefruit diet
16. fasting
17. vegetable cure
18. less salt
19. less sugar
20. less fat
21. less meat
22. more fluids
23. (more) biologic/nutritional products
24. more fresh vegetables and fruit
25. not on this chart

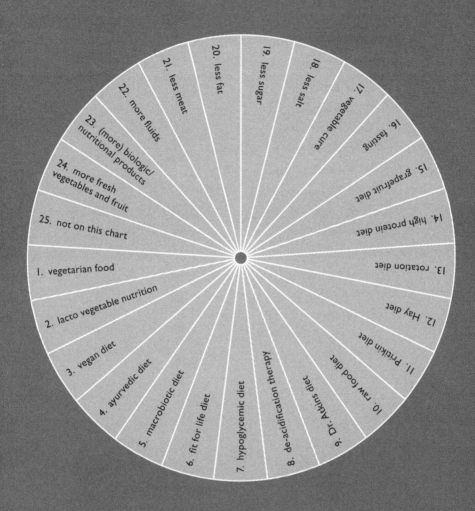

20. less fat
21. less meat
22. more fluids
23. (more) biologic/nutritional products
24. more fresh vegetables and fruit
25. not on this chart
1. vegetarian food
2. lacto vegetable nutrition
3. vegan diet
4. ayurvedic diet
5. macrobiotic diet
6. fit for life diet
7. hypoglycemic diet
8. de-acidification therapy
9. Dr. Atkins diet
10. raw food diet
11. Pritikin diet
12. Hay diet
13. rotation diet
14. high protein diet
15. grapefruit diet
16. fasting
17. vegetable cure
18. less salt
19. less sugar

Which kind of diet (or nutrition) should I avoid?

CHART 17

On which lifestyle habits should I focus?

1. I get too little rest at night
2. I relax too little
3. I don't get enough exercise
4. I get too little fresh air
5. I eat too few nutritious meals
6. I drink too much coffee
7. smoking
8. I drink too much alcohol
9. too many stimulants/depressants
10. I eat too many salty/fatty meals
11. I take too little time for myself
12. I take too little time for others
13. I feel way too responsible for my work
14. I feel way too responsible for others
15. not on this chart

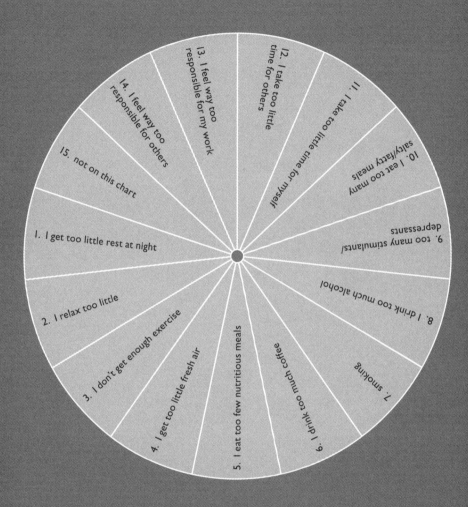

On which lifestyle habits should I focus?

The wheel contains the following segments:

1. I get too little rest at night
2. I relax too little
3. I don't get enough exercise
4. I get too little fresh air
5. I eat too few nutritious meals
6. I drink too much coffee
7. smoking
8. I drink too much alcohol
9. too many stimulants/depressants
10. I eat too many salty/fatty meals
11. I take too little time for myself
12. I take too little time for others
13. I feel way too responsible for my work
14. I feel way too responsible for others
15. not on this chart

CHART 18

I am too stressed. What is the reason for that?

1. too great a work load
2. worries (about money, etc.)
3. love-sickness
4. unexplainable fears/phobias
5. I ask too much of myself
6. I cannot plan my time efficiently
7. I get easily distracted from my work
8. I cannot relax
9. the problems of others
10. I have a problem saying no
11. I have too much responsibility
12. I don't dare ask for help
13. I can't stand criticism
14. I often make wrong decisions
15. not on this chart

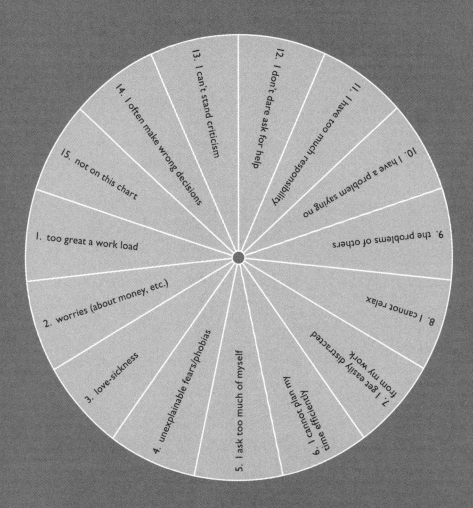

13. I can't stand criticism

12. I don't dare ask for help

11. I have too much responsibility

14. I often make wrong decisions

10. I have a problem saying no

15. not on this chart

9. the problems of others

1. too great a work load

8. I cannot relax

2. worries (about money, etc.)

7. I get easily distracted from my work

3. love-sickness

6. I cannot plan my time efficiently

4. unexplainable fears/phobias

5. I ask too much of myself

I am too stressed. What is the reason for that?

CHART 19

What kind of beauty care should I focus on?

1. daily hygiene
2. clothes—comfortable
3. clothes—sporty
4. clothes—fashionable
5. clothes—correct
6. hairstyle
7. nails
8. teeth
9. makeup
10. skin
11. perfume
12. jewelry
13. accessories
14. shoes
15. not on this chart

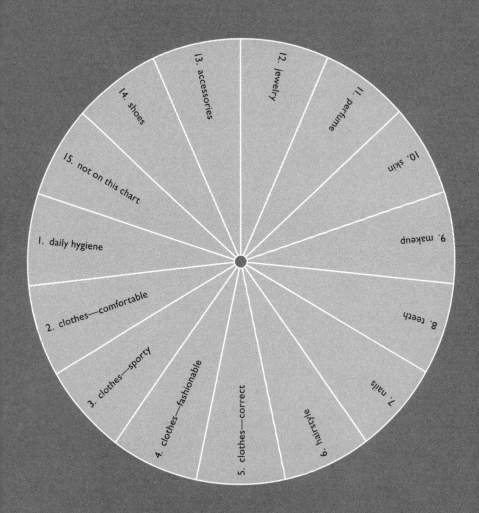

1. daily hygiene
2. clothes—comfortable
3. clothes—sporty
4. clothes—fashionable
5. clothes—correct
6. hairstyle
7. nails
8. teeth
9. makeup
10. skin
11. perfume
12. jewelry
13. accessories
14. shoes
15. not on this chart

What kind of beauty care should I focus on?

CHART 20

Which regular body care treatments are best for me?

1. hairstyle, haircut and styling
2. hairstyle, styling and color
3. cosmetic treatment
4. facial massage
5. body massage
6. beauty masks/face packs
7. nutritious masks/toners
8. solarium
9. sport massage
10. lymph drainage
11. manicure
12. pedicure
13. special skin care
14. careful makeup
15. not on this chart

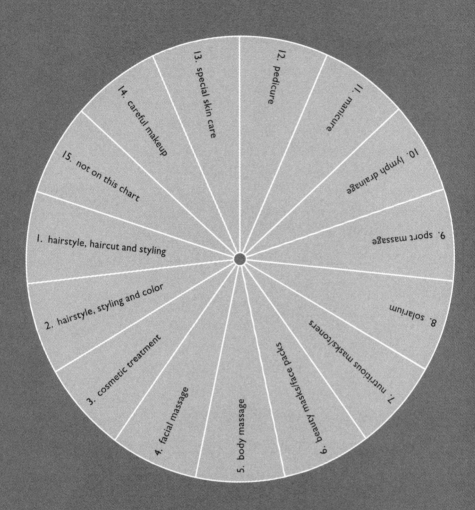

Which regular body care treatments are best for me?

13. special skin care

12. pedicure

14. careful makeup

11. manicure

15. not on this chart

10. lymph drainage

1. hairstyle, haircut and styling

9. sport massage

2. hairstyle, styling and color

8. solarium

3. cosmetic treatment

7. nutritious masks/toners

4. facial massage

6. beauty masks/face packs

5. body massage

CHART 21

Which kind of cleansing suits me best?

1. warm herbal bath—stimulating
2. warm herbal bath—relaxing
3. warm bath—without additives
4. lukewarm bath—without additives
5. showering (warm) for a long time
6. showering (lukewarm) for a long time
7. warm oil bath
8. warm bubble bath
9. short warm shower
10. short lukewarm shower
11. pouring water from a container
12. warm, cold rinsing
13. lukewarm, short rinsing
14. I do not prefer anything
15. not on this chart

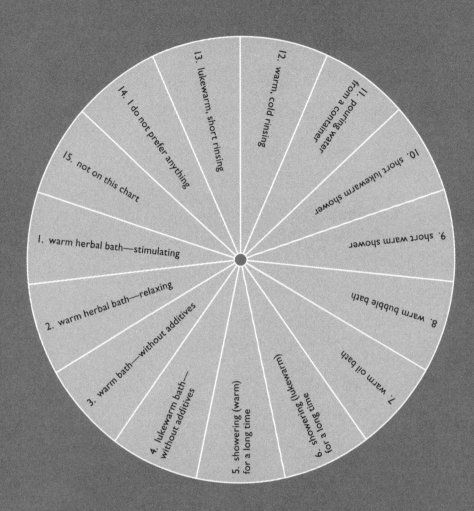

Which kind of cleansing suits me best?

1. warm herbal bath—stimulating
2. warm herbal bath—relaxing
3. warm bath—without additives
4. lukewarm bath—without additives
5. showering (warm) for a long time
6. showering (lukewarm) for a long time
7. warm oil bath
8. warm bubble bath
9. short warm shower
10. short lukewarm shower
11. pouring water from a container
12. warm; cold rinsing
13. lukewarm; short rinsing
14. I do not prefer anything
15. not on this chart

CHART 22

On which mental/psychological areas should I concentrate?

1. balanced energies
2. relaxation
3. energy
4. spirituality
5. enmeshment
6. self-confidence
7. inner growth
8. intellectual incentive
9. creative incentive
10. inspiration
11. stress
12. concentration
13. liveliness
14. self-observation
15. openness
16. flexibility
17. excitement
18. discipline
19. love
20. letting go
21. learning from mistakes
22. self-affirmation
23. motivation
24. forgiveness
25. not on this chart

SEE ALSO PENDULUM CHART 29

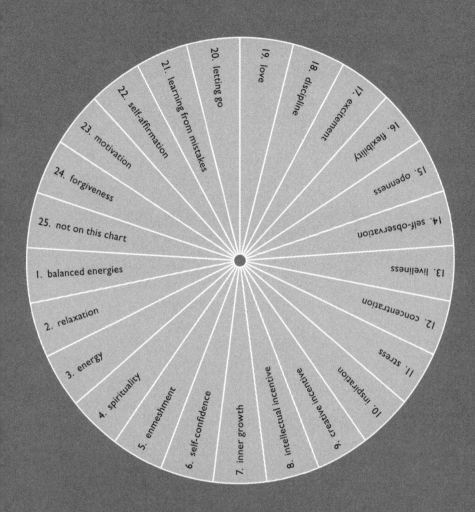

On which mental/psychological areas should I concentrate?

1. balanced energies
2. relaxation
3. energy
4. spirituality
5. enmeshment
6. self-confidence
7. inner growth
8. intellectual incentive
9. creative incentive
10. inspiration
11. stress
12. concentration
13. liveliness
14. self-observation
15. openness
16. flexibility
17. excitement
18. discipline
19. love
20. letting go
21. learning from mistakes
22. self-affirmation
23. motivation
24. forgiveness
25. not on this chart

CHART 23

On which physical areas should I concentrate?

1. immune system
2. circulation
3. heart
4. bladder and urinary tract
5. glands
6. skeleton
7. joints
8. nervous system
9. hair
10. skin and nails
11. sex organs
12. digestion (i.e. digestive organs)
13. lungs
14. muscles and tendons
15. connective tissue and cartilage
16. spine and cervical vertebra
17. eyesight
18. sense of touch
19. smell
20. taste
21. hearing
22. motor activity
23. teeth
24. energy balance
25. not on this chart

SEE ALSO PENDULUM CHART 28

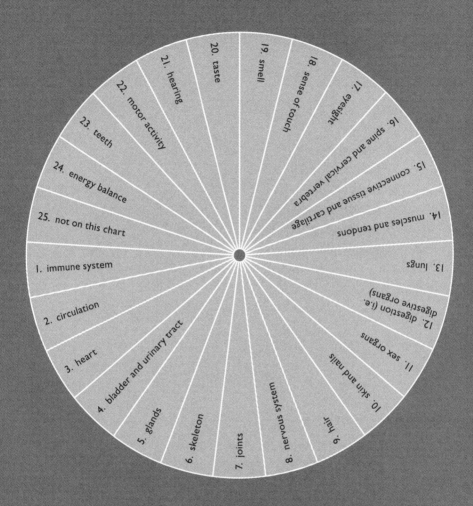

On which physical areas should I concentrate?

The wheel contains the following numbered segments:

1. immune system
2. circulation
3. heart
4. bladder and urinary tract
5. glands
6. skeleton
7. joints
8. nervous system
9. hair
10. skin and nails
11. sex organs
12. digestion (i.e. digestive organs)
13. lungs
14. muscles and tendons
15. connective tissue and cartilage
16. spine and cervical vertebra
17. eyesight
18. sense of touch
19. smell
20. taste
21. hearing
22. motor activity
23. teeth
24. energy balance
25. not on this chart

CHART 24

What kind of pain/infection should I focus on overcoming?

1. headaches
2. stomachaches
3. joint aches
4. neuralgia
5. muscle aches
6. sore throat
7. balding
8. ear infection
9. stomach infection/enteritis
10. bladder/urinary tract infection
11. infection of the airways
12. eye infection
13. skin allergy
14. gum disease
15. not on this chart

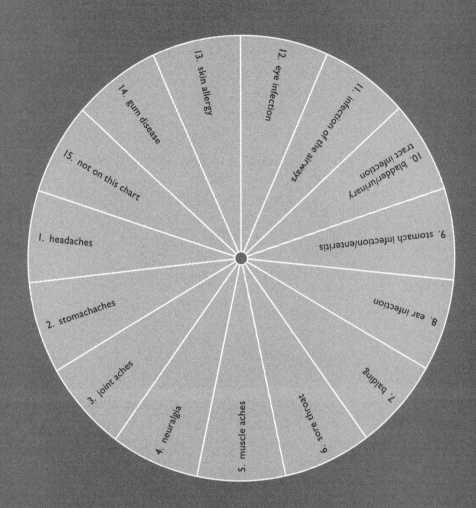

What kind of pain/infection should I focus on overcoming?

13. skin allergy
12. eye infection
14. gum disease
11. infection of the airways
15. not on this chart
10. bladder/urinary tract infection
1. headaches
9. stomach infection/enteritis
2. stomachaches
8. ear infection
3. joint aches
7. balding
4. neuralgia
6. sore throat
5. muscle aches

CHART 25

What physical conditions should I concentrate on overcoming?

1. sleepiness
2. hyperactivity
3. infections/inflammations
4. breathlessness
5. fatigue
6. excessive sweating
7. excessive blushing
8. allergies
9. poor concentration
10. high blood pressure
11. low blood pressure
12. no appetite
13. too great an appetite
14. muscle ache
15. not on this chart

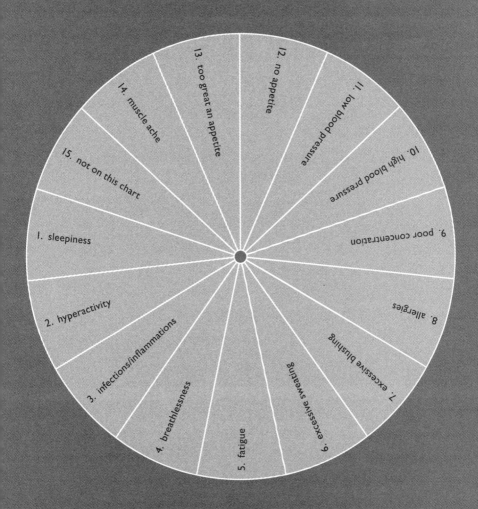

1. sleepiness
2. hyperactivity
3. infections/inflammations
4. breathlessness
5. fatigue
6. excessive sweating
7. excessive blushing
8. allergies
9. poor concentration
10. high blood pressure
11. low blood pressure
12. no appetite
13. too great an appetite
14. muscle ache
15. not on this chart

What physical conditions should I concentrate on overcoming?

CHART 26

Where in my body is the most important cause of my illness/suffering—#1?

1. cerebrum, nerve center
2. cerebral membrane
3. eyes
4. ears
5. nasal bone
6. jaw bone
7. tonsils
8. larynx
9. thyroid gland
10. air tube
11. shoulder joint
12. bronchia
13. right lung
14. liver
15. gall bladder
16. pancreas
17. colon, horizontal part
18. lower part of the aorta
19. inferior vena cava
20. colon, lower part
21. rectum
22. small intestine, winding part
23. appendix, front right
24. vermiform appendix
25. glands

PLEASE CONSULT YOUR DOCTOR SO THAT THE CORRECT DIAGNOSIS CAN BE MADE FOR THE PAINS YOU'RE EXPERIENCING.

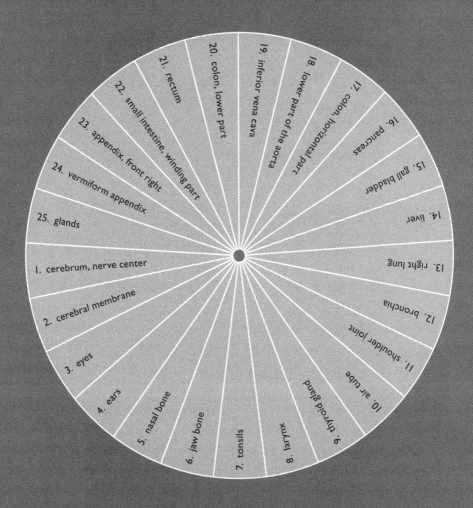

19. inferior vena cava
18. lower part of the aorta
17. colon, horizontal part
16. pancreas
15. gall bladder
14. liver
13. right lung
12. bronchia
11. shoulder joint
10. air tube
9. thyroid gland
8. larynx
7. tonsils
6. jaw bone
5. nasal bone
4. ears
3. eyes
2. cerebral membrane
1. cerebrum, nerve center
25. glands
24. vermiform appendix
23. appendix, front right
22. small intestine, winding part
21. rectum
20. colon, lower part

Where in my body is the most important cause of my illness/
suffering—#1?

CHART 27

Where in my body is the most important cause of my illness/ suffering—#2?

1. glands
2. circulation, arteries, and veins
3. ankle
4. hair
5. pituitary gland (hypophysis)
6. cerebellum
7. spinal cord (main nerve)
8. aorta
9. tip of the lung
10. breast gland (thymus gland)
11. left eye
12. esophagus
13. heart
14. stomach
15. elbow joint
16. spleen
17. kidneys
18. pelvis
19. urethra
20. hip joint
21. bladder
22. wrists
23. sex organs
24. knee joint
25. not on this chart

PLEASE CONSULT YOUR DOCTOR SO THAT THE CORRECT DIAGNOSIS CAN BE MADE FOR THE PAINS YOU'RE EXPERIENCING.

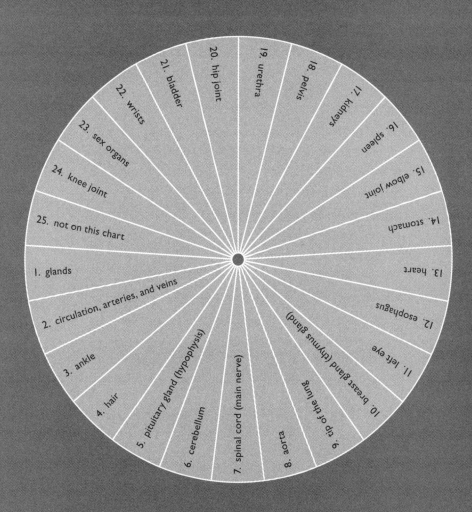

*Where in my body is the most important cause of my illness/
suffering—#2?*

CHART 28

What important physical factor is the cause of my illness/suffering?

1. physical overstrain
2. lack of physical activity
3. lack of vital nutrients
4. poor absorption of vital nutrients
5. poor detoxification
6. too little water
7. too little fresh air
8. poor posture/not enough exercise
9. chronic (unknown) infection
10. unknown malfunction
11. shallow breathing
12. disturbing radiation
13. energetic imbalance
14. abuse of medications
15. not on this chart

PLEASE CONSULT YOUR DOCTOR SO THAT THE CORRECT DIAGNOSIS CAN BE MADE FOR THE PAIN YOU'RE EXPERIENCING.

SEE ALSO PENDULUM CHART 23

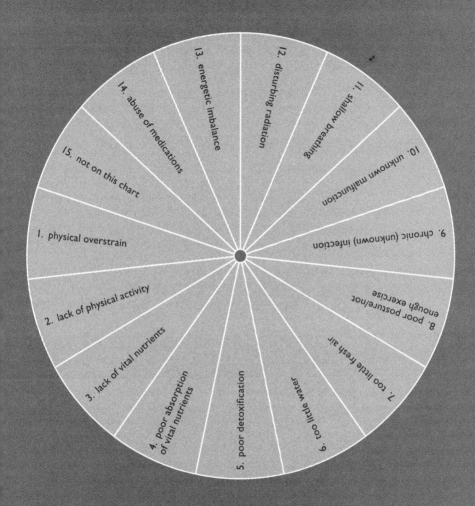

1. physical overstrain
2. lack of physical activity
3. lack of vital nutrients
4. poor absorption of vital nutrients
5. poor detoxification
6. too little water
7. too little fresh air
8. poor posture/not enough exercise
9. chronic (unknown) infection
10. unknown malfunction
11. shallow breathing
12. disturbing radiation
13. energetic imbalance
14. abuse of medications
15. not on this chart

What important physical factor is the cause of my illness/suffering?

CHART 29

What important mental factor is the cause of my illness/suffering?

1. acute worry
2. chronic worry (love sickness, grief)
3. fear of the unknown
4. fear of being abandoned
5. too little self-esteem
6. too little confidence
7. the feeling of not being appreciated
8. jealousy or envy
9. unprocessed rage
10. despair
11. suppressed feelings
12. feelings of hopelessness
13. panic
14. stress
15. not on this chart

PLEASE CONSULT YOUR DOCTOR SO THAT THE CORRECT DIAGNOSIS CAN BE MADE FOR THE KIND OF PAIN YOU'RE EXPERIENCING.

SEE ALSO PENDULUM CHART 22

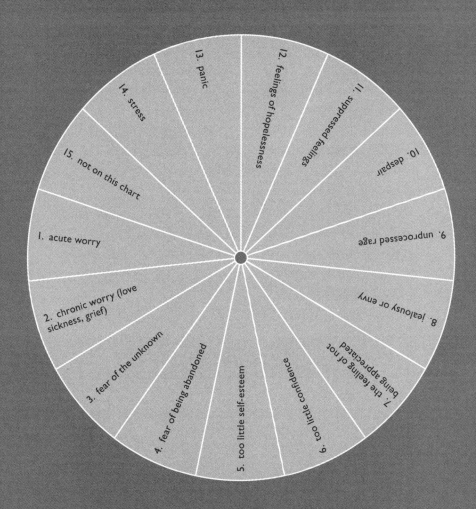

1. acute worry
2. chronic worry (love sickness, grief)
3. fear of the unknown
4. fear of being abandoned
5. too little self-esteem
6. too little confidence
7. the feeling of not being appreciated
8. jealousy or envy
9. unprocessed rage
10. despair
11. suppressed feeling
12. feelings of hopelessness
13. panic
14. stress
15. not on this chart

What important mental factor is the cause of my illness/suffering?

CHART 30

My (poor) condition is, among other things, influenced by:

1. poor nutrition
2. acute infection (bacterial/ viral)
3. chronic infection (bacterial/viral)
4. accident/injury
5. inherited condition
6. allergy
7. too strict a diet
8. fungal infection
9. parasites
10. traumatic experiences
11. repressed emotions
12. unprocessed experiences
13. unprocessed emotions
14. ignored injury
15. protracted infection
16. too many poisonous substances
17. too many toxins from environment
18. taking medications (currently)
19. taking medications (in the past)
20. proper behavioral patterns
21. adapted behavioral patterns
22. lack of sunlight
23. proper way of thinking
24. adapted way of thinking
25. not on this chart

PLEASE CONSULT YOUR DOCTOR SO THAT THE CORRECT DIAGNOSIS CAN BE MADE FOR THE PAIN YOU'RE EXPERIENCING.

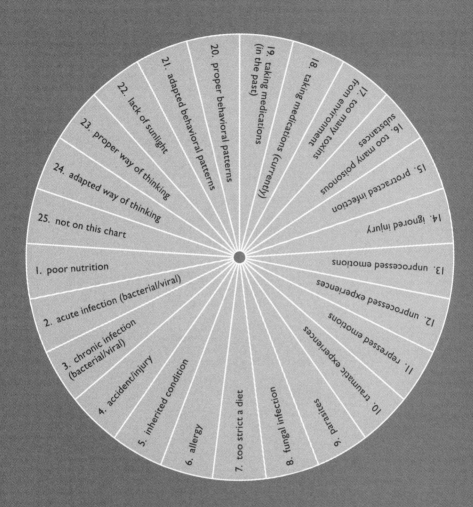

My (poor) condition is, among other things, influenced by:

The following labels appear around the wheel:

19. taking medications (in the past)
20. proper behavioral patterns
21. adapted behavioral patterns
22. lack of sunlight
23. proper way of thinking
24. adapted way of thinking
25. not on this chart
1. poor nutrition
2. acute infection (bacterial/viral)
3. chronic infection (bacterial/viral)
4. accident/injury
5. inherited condition
6. allergy
7. too strict a diet
8. fungal infection
9. parasites
10. traumatic experiences
11. repressed emotions
12. unprocessed experiences
13. unprocessed emotions
14. ignored injury
15. protracted infection
16. too many poisonous substances
17. too many toxins from environment
18. taking medications (currently)

CHART 31

To what substances am I allergic?

1. cat hair
2. dog hair
3. rodent hair, dust
4. bird mites, dust
5. bee stings
6. wasp stings
7. tick bites
8. mosquito bites
9. flea bites
10. house mites
11. hay and grain dust
12. pollen
13. poison ivy
14. poison oak
15. not on this chart

SEE ALSO PENDULUM CHARTS 12, 32, 55, 109, 119

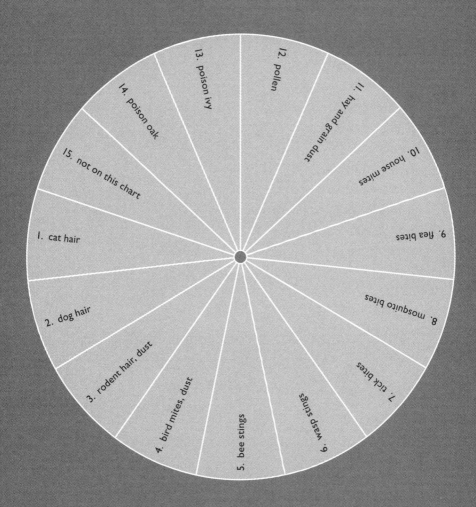

14. poison oak
13. poison ivy
12. pollen
11. hay and grain dust
10. house mites
9. flea bites
15. not on this chart
1. cat hair
2. dog hair
3. rodent hair, dust
4. bird mites, dust
5. bee stings
6. wasp stings
7. tick bites
8. mosquito bites

To what substances am I allergic?

CHART 32

To which kind of substances/circumstances am I allergic?

1. house dust
2. synthetic dyes
3. synthetic varnishes
4. car exhaust
5. ammonia
6. formaldehyde
7. insecticides/artificial fertilizer
8. underground power currents
9. electromagnetic fields
10. too much direct sunlight
11. chloride
12. salt
13. water
14. soap
15. not on this chart

SEE ALSO PENDULUM CHARTS 12, 31, 55, 109, 119

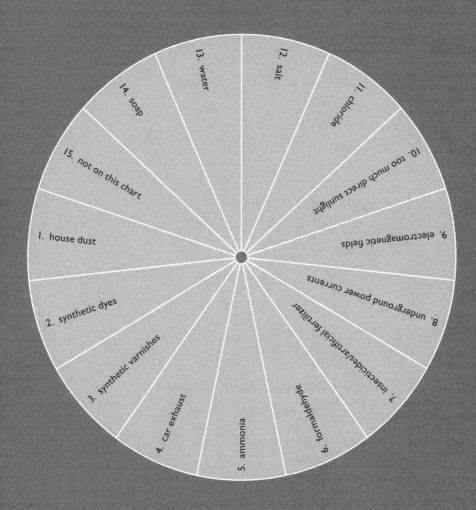

To which kind of substances/circumstances am I allergic?

1. house dust
2. synthetic dyes
3. synthetic varnishes
4. car exhaust
5. ammonia
6. formaldehyde
7. insecticides/artificial fertilizer
8. underground power currents
9. electromagnetic fields
10. too much direct sunlight
11. chloride
12. salt
13. water
14. soap
15. not on this chart

CHART 33

Which of my seven chakras is blocked or should be cleansed, and how much?

1. first chakra—a little
2. second chakra—a little
3. third chakra—a little
4. fourth chakra—a little
5. fifth chakra—a little
6. sixth chakra—a little
7. seventh chakra—a little
8. first chakra—a great deal
9. second chakra—a great deal
10. third chakra—a great deal
11. fourth chakra—a great deal
12. fifth chakra—a great deal
13. sixth chakra— a great deal
14. seventh chakra—a great deal
15. none of the chakras

POSE THIS QUESTION, IF NECESSARY, SEVEN TIMES!

IN LITERATURE ABOUT THE CHAKRAS, YOU WILL FIND SPECIAL
EXERCISES AND REMEDIES.

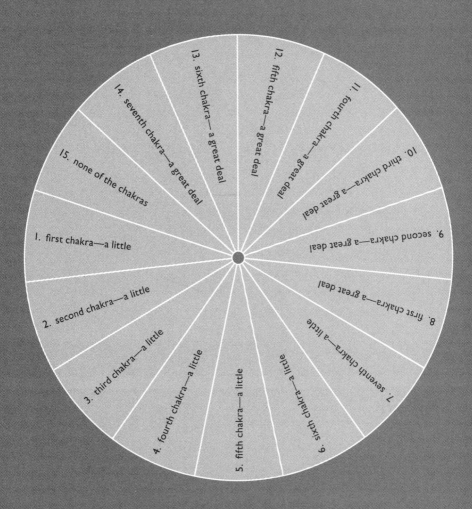

1. first chakra—a little
2. second chakra—a little
3. third chakra—a little
4. fourth chakra—a little
5. fifth chakra—a little
6. sixth chakra—a little
7. seventh chakra—a little
8. first chakra—a great deal
9. second chakra—a great deal
10. third chakra—a great deal
11. fourth chakra—a great deal
12. fifth chakra—a great deal
13. sixth chakra—a great deal
14. seventh chakra—a great deal
15. none of the chakras

*Which of my seven chakras is blocked or should be cleansed,
and how much?*

CHART 34

Which of my seven chakras is dominant?

1. first chakra—a little
2. second chakra—a little
3. third chakra—a little
4. fourth chakra—a little
5. fifth chakra—a little
6. sixth chakra—a little
7. seventh chakra—a little
8. first chakra—a great deal
9. second chakra—a great deal
10. third chakra—a great deal
11. fourth chakra—a great deal
12. fifth chakra—a great deal
13. sixth chakra— a great deal
14. seventh chakra—a great deal
15. none of the chakras

IN LITERATURE ABOUT THE CHAKRAS, YOU'LL FIND SPECIAL EXERCISES AND REMEDIES.

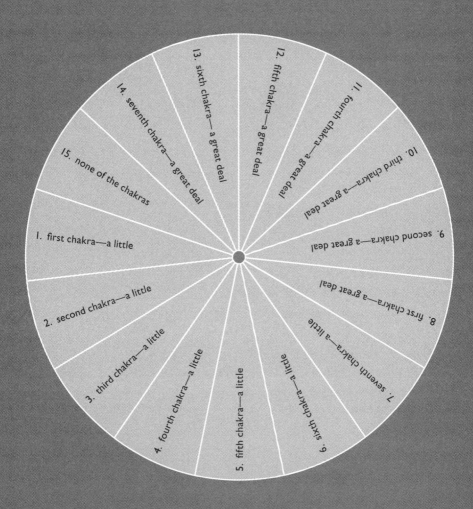

1. first chakra—a little
2. second chakra—a little
3. third chakra—a little
4. fourth chakra—a little
5. fifth chakra—a little
6. sixth chakra—a little
7. seventh chakra—a little
8. first chakra—a great deal
9. second chakra—a great deal
10. third chakra—a great deal
11. fourth chakra—a great deal
12. fifth chakra—a great deal
13. sixth chakra—a great deal
14. seventh chakra—a great deal
15. none of the chakras

Which of my seven chakras is dominant?

CHART 35

Which of my main meridians is blocked?

1. liver meridian
2. heart meridian
3. spleen-pancreas meridian
4. lung meridian
5. kidney meridian
6. circulation-sex meridian
7. gall bladder meridian
8. small intestine meridian
9. stomach meridian
10. colon meridian
11. bladder meridian
12. triple-warmer meridian
13. conception meridian
14. pericardial meridian
15. not on this chart

IN LITERATURE ABOUT MERIDIANS, YOU'LL FIND SPECIAL
EXERCISES AND REMEDIES.

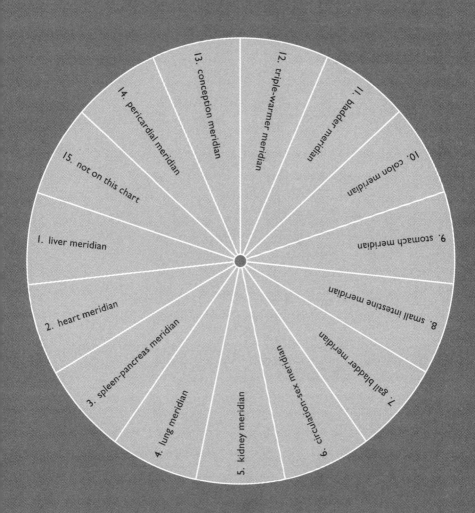

Which of my main meridians is blocked?

CHART 36

What attitudes are involved with my chakra/meridian blockage?

1. I "forgive and forget" with great effort
2. I think in terms of "black and white"
3. I think too theoretically
4. I place my own interests last
5. I act only out of self-interest
6. I reject aspects of myself
7. I do not want to have responsibility
8. I want to have it my way . . .
9. I can't accept things "just like that"
10. I suffer from "helpfulness syndrome"
11. my prejudice(s) get in my way
12. I deceive myself
13. I want to suffer (unconsciously)
14. I neglect my feelings
15. not on this chart

SEE ALSO PENDULUM CHARTS 65 TO 71

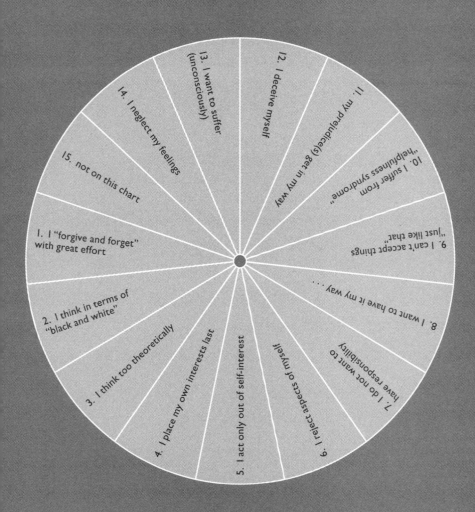

1. I "forgive and forget" with great effort
2. I think in terms of "black and white"
3. I think too theoretically
4. I place my own interests last
5. I act only out of self-interest
6. I reject aspects of myself
7. I do not want to have responsibility
8. I want to have it my way . . .
9. I can't accept things "just like that"
10. I suffer from "helpfulness syndrome"
11. my prejudice(s) get in my way
12. I deceive myself
13. I want to suffer (unconsciously)
14. I neglect my feelings
15. not on this chart

What attitudes are involved with my chakra/meridian blockage?

CHART 37

What nutritional supplements should I take?

1. cod liver oil
2. brewer's yeast
3. spirulina
4. kelp
5. royal jelly
6. bee pollen
7. ginkgo biloba
8. fibers
9. wheat germ
10. garlic (capsules)
11. lecithin
12. jojoba
13. coenzyme Q-10
14. alpha lipoic acid
15. not on this chart

CONSULT YOUR DOCTOR BEFORE TAKING NUTRITIONAL
SUPPLEMENTS!

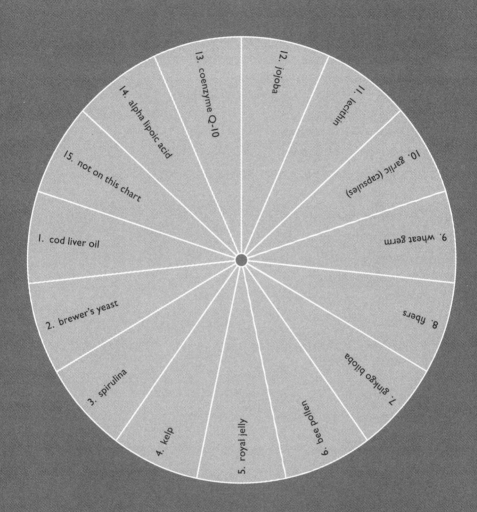

What nutritional supplements should I take?

1. cod liver oil
2. brewer's yeast
3. spirulina
4. kelp
5. royal jelly
6. bee pollen
7. ginkgo biloba
8. fibers
9. wheat germ
10. garlic (capsules)
11. lecithin
12. jojoba
13. coenzyme Q-10
14. alpha lipoic acid
15. not on this chart

CHART 38

What antioxidants should I take?

1. selenium
2. vitamin C
3. vitamin E
4. superoxide dismutase (S.O.D.)
5. shitake mushrooms
6. reishi mushrooms (Ling Ching)
7. beta-carotene
8. germanium
9. glutathione
10. gammalin acid
11. coenzyme Q-10
12. grape seed
13. alpha lipoic acid
14. lycopene
15. not on this chart

CONSULT YOUR DOCTOR BEFORE TAKING ANTIOXIDANTS!

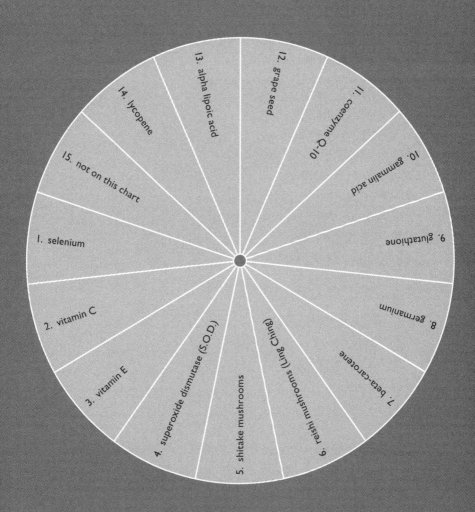

What antioxidants should I take?

CHART 39

What cell salts should I take?

1. potassium phosphate
2. potassium sulphate
3. potassium chloride
4. sodium sulphate
5. sodium chloride
6. calcium sulphate
7. calcium phosphate
8. calcium fluoride
9. magnesium phosphate
10. sodium phosphate
11. iron phosphate
12. silica
13. none
14. several
15. not on this chart

CONSULT YOUR DOCTOR BEFORE TAKING CELL SALTS!

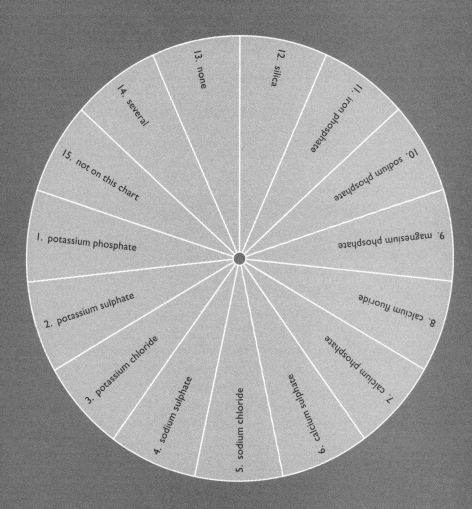

What cell salts should I take?

CHART 40

What medicinal herbs should I use—#1?

1. agrimony	14. laserwort
2. scullcap	15. aloe vera
3. witch hazel	16. dead nettle,
4. bayberry	white
5. borage	17. goldenseal
6. betony	18. yarrow
7. chicory	19. milk thistle
8. scotch broom	20. milkweed
9. mugwort	21. saw palmetto
10. nettle, stinging	22. goldenrod
11. speedwell	23. motherwort
12. southernwood	24. allheal
13. lemon balm	25. not on this chart

CONSULT YOUR DOCTOR OR MEDICAL PRACTITIONER FOR THE CORRECT APPLICATION OF MEDICINAL HERBS.

IN LITERATURE ABOUT MEDICINAL HERBS, YOU WILL FIND THE CORRECT APPLICATION (FOR EXAMPLE, INTERNAL OR EXTERNAL USE, ONLY LEAVES, STEMS, OR ROOTS, ETC.).

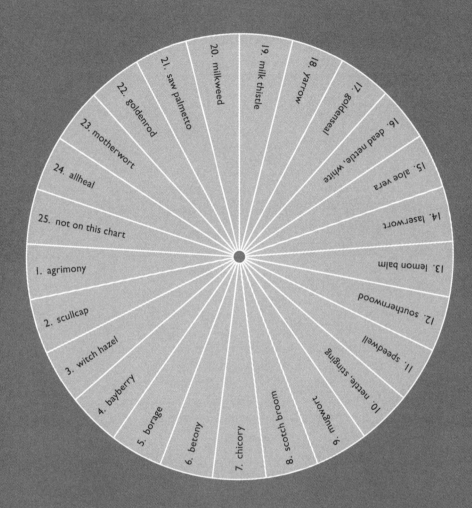

1. agrimony
2. scullcap
3. witch hazel
4. bayberry
5. borage
6. betony
7. chicory
8. scotch broom
9. mugwort
10. nettle, stinging
11. speedwell
12. southernwood
13. lemon balm
14. laserwort
15. aloe vera
16. dead nettle, white
17. goldenseal
18. yarrow
19. milk thistle
20. milkweed
21. saw palmetto
22. goldenrod
23. motherwort
24. allheal
25. not on this chart

What medicinal herbs should I use—#1?

CHART 41

What medicinal herbs should I use—#2?

1. shepherd's purse
2. ground ivy
3. echinacea
4. ginger
5. hyssop
6. lupine
7. juniper berries
8. mallow
9. chamomile, German
10. chamomile, bolegold
11. angelica
12. blue cohosh
13. coltsfoot
14. garlic
15. willow herb
16. French sorrel
17. laceflower
18. stoneroot
19. maitake
20. gotu kola
21. tamarind
22. feverfew
23. meadowsweet
24. eyebright
25. not on this chart

CONSULT YOUR DOCTOR OR MEDICAL PRACTITIONER FOR THE CORRECT APPLICATION OF MEDICINAL HERBS.

IN LITERATURE ABOUT MEDICINAL HERBS YOU'LL FIND THE CORRECT APPLICATION (FOR EXAMPLE, INTERNAL OR EXTERNAL USE, ONLY LEAVES, STEMS, OR ROOTS, ETC.).

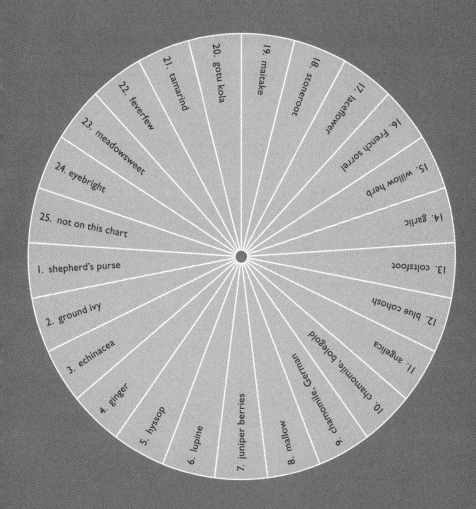

1. shepherd's purse
2. ground ivy
3. echinacea
4. ginger
5. hyssop
6. lupine
7. juniper berries
8. mallow
9. chamomile, German
10. chamomile, bolegold
11. angelica
12. blue cohosh
13. coltsfoot
14. garlic
15. willow herb
16. French sorrel
17. laceflower
18. stoneroot
19. maitake
20. gotu kola
21. tamarind
22. feverfew
23. meadowsweet
24. eyebright
25. not on this chart

What medicinal herbs should I use—#2?

CHART 42

What medicinal herbs should I use—#3?

1. nasturtium
2. peppermint
3. psyllium
4. schisandra
5. ramsons
6. wormwood
7. Solomon's seal
8. California poppy
9. boneset
10. black-eyed Susan
11. figwort (do not use while pregnant)
12. St John's Wort
13. evening primrose
14. thyme, wild
15. not on this chart

CONSULT YOUR DOCTOR OR MEDICAL PRACTITIONER FOR THE
CORRECT APPLICATION OF MEDICINAL HERBS.

IN LITERATURE ABOUT MEDICINAL HERBS, YOU'LL FIND THE
CORRECT APPLICATION (FOR EXAMPLE, INTERNAL OR EXTERNAL
USE, ONLY LEAVES, STEMS, OR ROOTS, ETC.).

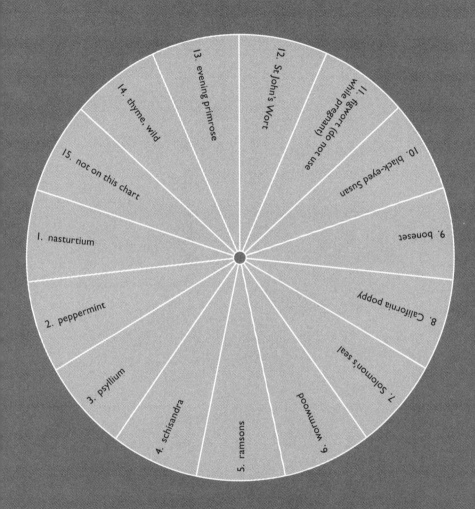

What medicinal herbs should I use—#3?

13. evening primrose

12. St John's Wort

11. figwort (do not use while pregnant)

10. black-eyed Susan

9. boneset

8. California poppy

7. Solomon's seal

6. wormwood

5. ramsons

4. schisandra

3. psyllium

2. peppermint

1. nasturtium

15. not on this chart

14. thyme, wild

CHART 43

What medicinal herbs should I use—#4?

1. valerian
2. fennel
3. vervain
4. pokeroot
5. chickweed
6. lady's-mantle
7. common plantain
8. plantain, ribgrass
9. arnica
10. burdock
11. ginkgo
12. coneflower, yellow
13. French sorrel
14. mullein
15. not on this chart

CONSULT YOUR DOCTOR OR MEDICAL PRACTITIONER FOR THE CORRECT APPLICATION OF MEDICINAL HERBS.

IN LITERATURE ABOUT MEDICINAL HERBS, YOU'LL FIND THE APPROPRIATE APPLICATION (FOR INSTANCE, INNER OR OUTER USE, ONLY LEAVES, STEMS, OR ROOTS, ETC.).

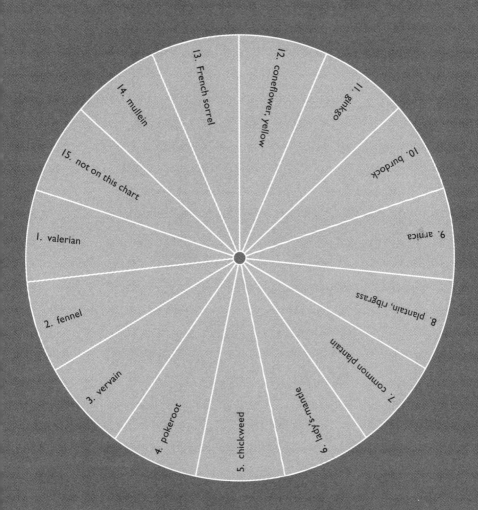

What medicinal herbs should I use—#4?

CHART 44

Which essential oil is most useful to me—#1?

1. tagetes
2. anise
3. allspice
4. basil
5. benzoin
6. bergamot
7. birch
8. cajeput
9. cedarwood
10. cypress
11. rockrose
12. lemon
13. citronella

14. pine, scotch
15. dill
16. bay rum
17. cassia
18. yarrow
19. angelica
20. eucalyptus
21. galbanum
22. ginger root
23. geranium
24. fir
25. not on this chart

CONSULT YOUR DOCTOR OR MEDICAL PRACTITIONER FOR THE CORRECT APPLICATION OF ESSENTIAL OILS.

IN LITERATURE ABOUT ESSENTIAL OILS, YOU'LL FIND THE CORRECT APPLICATION.

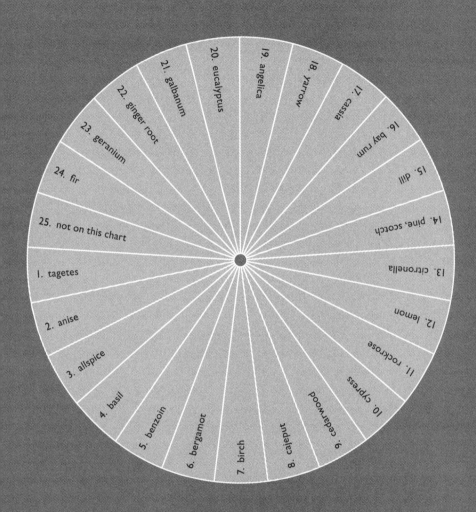

Which essential oil is most useful to me—#1?

CHART 45

Which essential oil is most useful to me—#2?

1. Oregon breeze
2. clary sage
3. hyssop
4. jasmine
5. juniper berry
6. lantana camara
7. camphor, white
8. chamomile, German
9. chamomile, Roman
10. cinnamon
11. cardamom
12. pennyroyal
13. opoponax wildcrafted
14. coriander
15. clove
16. geranium bourbon
17. bay laurel
18. wintergreen
19. lavender
20. lavendin
21. lemongrass
22. lime
23. linden blossom
24. litsea
25. not on this chart

CONSULT YOUR DOCTOR OR MEDICAL PRACTITIONER FOR THE CORRECT APPLICATION OF ESSENTIAL OILS.

IN LITERATURE ABOUT ESSENTIAL OILS YOU'LL FIND THE CORRECT APPLICATION.

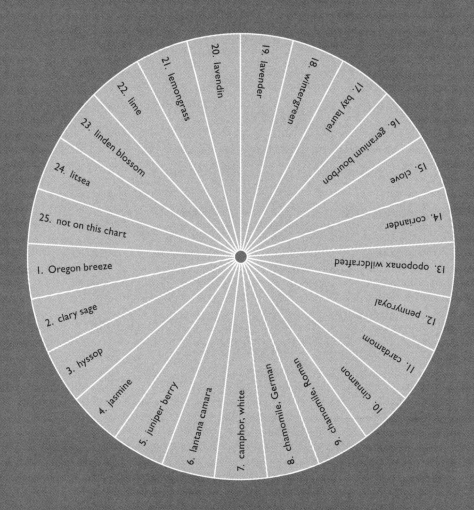

Which essential oil is most useful to me—#2?

1. Oregon breeze
2. clary sage
3. hyssop
4. jasmine
5. juniper berry
6. lantana camara
7. camphor, white
8. chamomile, German
9. chamomile, Roman
10. cinnamon
11. cardamom
12. pennyroyal
13. opoponax wildcrafted
14. coriander
15. clove
16. geranium bourbon
17. bay laurel
18. wintergreen
19. lavender
20. lavendin
21. lemongrass
22. lime
23. linden blossom
24. litsea
25. not on this chart

CHART 46

Which essential oil is most useful to me—#3?

1. mandarin
2. marjoram
3. ravensara
4. verbena
5. myrrh
6. peppermint
7. scotch pine
8. valerian root
9. myrtle
10. spikenard
11. sage
12. niaouli
13. nutmeg

14. palmarosa
15. patchouli
16. pepper, black
17. Peruvian balsam
18. parsley
19. petitgrain
20. rosemary verbenone
21. grapefruit
22. rose
23. rosemary
24. rosewood
25. not on this chart

CONSULT YOUR DOCTOR OR MEDICAL PRACTITIONER FOR THE
CORRECT APPLICATION OF ESSENTIAL OILS.

IN LITERATURE ABOUT ESSENTIAL OILS, YOU'LL FIND THE
CORRECT APPLICATION.

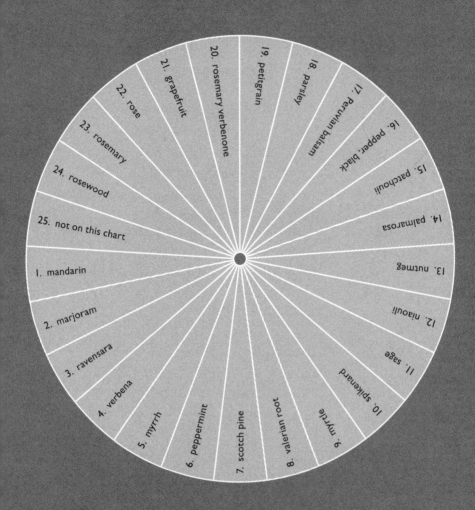

Which essential oil is most useful to me—#3?

1. mandarin
2. marjoram
3. ravensara
4. verbena
5. myrrh
6. peppermint
7. scotch pine
8. valerian root
9. myrtle
10. spikenard
11. sage
12. niaouli
13. nutmeg
14. palmarosa
15. patchouli
16. pepper, black
17. Peruvian balsam
18. parsley
19. petitgrain
20. rosemary verbenone
21. grapefruit
22. rose
23. rosemary
24. rosewood
25. not on this chart

CHART 47

Which essential oil is most useful to me—#4?

1. sage dalmation
2. thyme borneol ecocert
3. sandalwood
4. cinnamon bark
5. bitter orange
6. orange, sweet
7. neroli
8. spruce
9. fir needle
10. oregano
11. helichrysum
12. spearmint
13. tea tree, common
14. thyme
15. tangerine
16. tuberose
17. cedarwood, Virginia
18. fennel
19. eucalyptus citriodora
20. eucalyptus radiata
21. vetiver
22. violet leaf
23. carrot seed
24. ylang-ylang
25. not on this chart

CONSULT YOUR DOCTOR OR MEDICAL PRACTITIONER FOR THE CORRECT APPLICATION OF ESSENTIAL OILS.

IN LITERATURE ABOUT ESSENTIAL OILS YOU'LL FIND THE CORRECT APPLICATION.

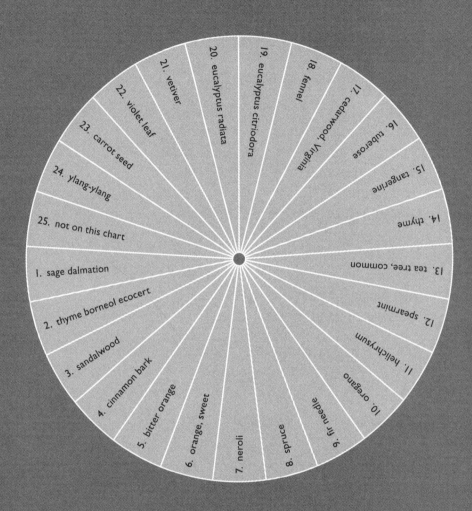

1. sage dalmation
2. thyme borneol ecocert
3. sandalwood
4. cinnamon bark
5. bitter orange
6. orange, sweet
7. neroli
8. spruce
9. fir needle
10. oregano
11. helichrysum
12. spearmint
13. tea tree, common
14. thyme
15. tangerine
16. tuberose
17. cedarwood, Virginia
18. fennel
19. eucalyptus citriodora
20. eucalyptus radiata
21. vetiver
22. violet leaf
23. carrot seed
24. ylang-ylang
25. not on this chart

Which essential oil is most useful to me—#4?

CHART 48

What Bach flowers should I use—#1?

1. agrimony	14. heather
2. aspen	15. holly
3. beech	16. honeysuckle
4. centaury	17. hornbeam
5. cerato	18. impatiens
6. cherry plum	19. larch
7. chestnut bud	20. mimulus
8. chicory	21. mustard
9. clematis	22. oak
10. crab apple	23. olive
11. elm	24. pine
12. gentian	25. not on this chart
13. gorse	

IN LITERATURE ABOUT BACH FLOWER THERAPY YOU'LL FIND THE
CORRECT APPLICATION.

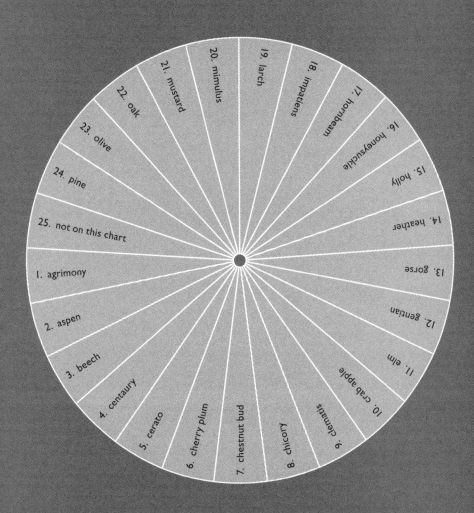

What Bach flowers should I use—#1?

CHART 49

What Bach flowers should I use—#2?

1. red chestnut
2. rockrose
3. rock water
4. scleranthus
5. star of Bethlehem
6. sweet chestnut
7. vervain
8. vine
9. walnut
10. water violet
11. white chestnut
12. wild oak
13. wild rose
14. willow
15. not on this chart

IN LITERATURE ABOUT BACH FLOWER THERAPY, YOU'LL FIND THE CORRECT APPLICATION.

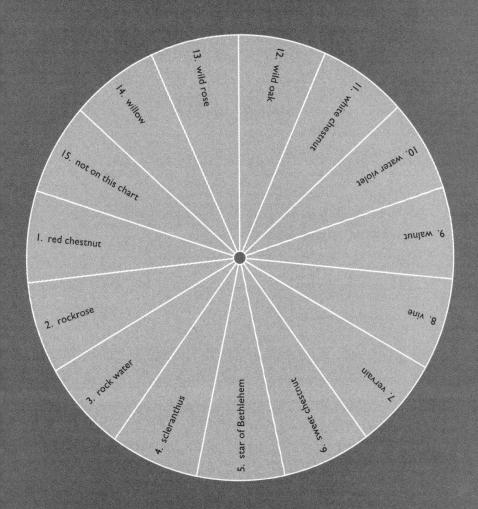

What Bach flowers should I use—#2?

CHART 50

Which stones, crystals, or minerals are of greatest use to me—#1?

1. carbonates
2. fluorspar
3. oxides: chalcedony group
4. oxides: corundum group
5. oxides: quartz group
6. diverse oxides
7. silicates: tourmaline group
8. silicates: beryl group
9. silicates: garnet group
10. silicates: jade group
11. diverse silicates
12. sulfates: feldspar group
13. diverse sulfates
14. precious stones of organic origin
15. not on this chart

ATTENTION: STONES, CRYSTALS, AND MINERALS ARE FOR
EXTERNAL USE ONLY!

LITERATURE ABOUT STONES, CRYSTALS, AND MINERALS PROVIDES
DETAILED INSIGHT INTO THEIR CORRECT APPLICATION.

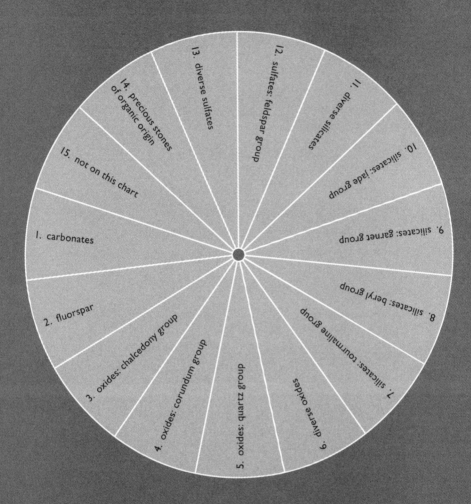

Which stones, crystals, or minerals are of greatest use to me—#1?

CHART 51

Which stones, crystals, or minerals are of greatest use to me—#2?

1. agate (oxide: chalcedony)
2. cornelian (oxide: chalcedony, quartz)
3. chrysoprase (oxide: chalcedony)
4. heliotrope (oxide: chalcedony)
5. jasper (oxide: chalcedony)
6. onyx (oxide: chalcedony)
7. sardonyx (oxide: chalcedony)
8. blue chalcedony (oxide: chalcedony)
9. ruby (oxide: corundum)
10. sapphire (oxide: corundum)
11. citrine (oxide: corundum)
12. amethyst (oxide: quartz)
13. cat's eye (oxide: quartz)
14. falcon's-eye (oxide: quartz)
15. smoky quartz (oxide: quartz)
16. aventurine (oxide: quartz)
17. rock crystal (oxide: quartz)
18. rose quartz (oxide: quartz)
19. magnetite (oxide)
20. obsidian (oxide)
21. opal (oxide)
22. hematite (oxide)
23. jadeite (silicates: jade group)
24. nephrite (silicates: jade group)
25. not on this chart

ATTENTION: STONES, CRYSTALS, AND MINERALS ARE FOR EXTERNAL USE ONLY!

LITERATURE ABOUT STONES, CRYSTALS, AND MINERALS PROVIDES DETAILED INSIGHT INTO THEIR CORRECT APPLICATION.

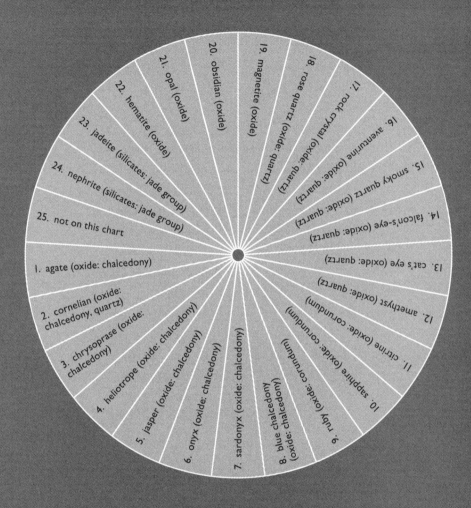

1. agate (oxide: chalcedony)
2. cornelian (oxide: chalcedony, quartz)
3. chrysoprase (oxide: chalcedony)
4. heliotrope (oxide: chalcedony)
5. jasper (oxide: chalcedony)
6. onyx (oxide: chalcedony)
7. sardonyx (oxide: chalcedony)
8. blue chalcedony (oxide: chalcedony)
9. ruby (oxide: corundum)
10. sapphire (oxide: corundum)
11. citrine (oxide: quartz)
12. amethyst (oxide: quartz)
13. cat's eye (oxide: quartz)
14. falcon's-eye (oxide: quartz)
15. smoky quartz (oxide: quartz)
16. aventurine (oxide: quartz)
17. rock crystal (oxide: quartz)
18. rose quartz (oxide: quartz)
19. magnetite (oxide)
20. obsidian (oxide)
21. opal (oxide)
22. hematite (oxide)
23. jadeite (silicates: jade group)
24. nephrite (silicates: jade group)
25. not on this chart

Which stones, crystals, or minerals are of greatest use to me—#2?

CHART 52

Which stones, crystals, or minerals are of greatest use to me—#3?

1. indicolite (silicates: tourmaline group)
2. rubellite (silicates: tourmaline group)
3. black tourmaline
4. verdelith (silicates: tourmaline group)
5. watermelon tourmaline
6. beryl (silicates: beryl group)
7. aquamarine (silicates: beryl group)
8. heliodor (silicates: beryl group)
9. morganite (silicates: beryl group)
10. emerald (silicates: beryl group)
11. garnet (silicates: garnet group)
12. almandine (silicates: garnet group)
13. pyrope (silicates: garnet group)
14. uvarovite (silicates: garnet group)
15. apophyllite (silicate)
16. charoit (silicate)
17. lapis lazuli (silicate)
18. olivine, peridot, and chrysolite
19. rhodonite (silicate)
20. sodalite (silicate)
21. stilbite (silicate)
22. sugilite (silicate)
23. topaz (silicate)
24. zircon (silicate)
25. not on this chart

ATTENTION: STONES, CRYSTALS, AND MINERALS ARE FOR EXTERNAL USE ONLY!

LITERATURE ABOUT STONES, CRYSTALS, AND MINERALS PROVIDES DETAILED INSIGHT INTO THEIR CORRECT APPLICATION.

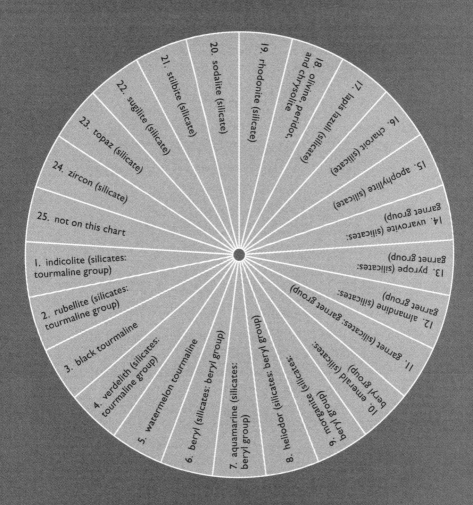

Which stones, crystals, or minerals are of greatest use to me—#3?

The wheel, reading clockwise from top, contains:

19. rhodonite (silicate)
18. olivine, and chrysolite and peridot,
17. lapis lazuli (silicate)
16. charoit (silicate)
15. apophyllite (silicate)
14. uvarovite (silicates: garnet group)
13. pyrope (silicates: garnet group)
12. almandine (silicates: garnet group)
11. garnet (silicates: garnet group)
10. emerald (silicates: beryl group)
9. morganite (silicates: beryl group)
8. heliodor (silicates: beryl group)
7. aquamarine (silicates: beryl group)
6. beryl (silicates: beryl group)
5. watermelon tourmaline
4. verdelith (silicates: tourmaline group)
3. black tourmaline
2. rubellite (silicates: tourmaline group)
1. indicolite (silicates: tourmaline group)
25. not on this chart
24. zircon (silicate)
23. topaz (silicate)
22. sugilite (silicate)
21. stilbite (silicate)
20. sodalite (silicate)

CHART 53

Which stones, crystals, or minerals are of greatest use to me—#4?

1. magnesite (carbonate)
2. malachite (carbonate)
3. dialogite (carbonate)
4. pyrite (sulfate)
5. turquoise (sulfate)
6. amazonite (sulfate: feldspar group)
7. labradorite (sulfate: feldspar group)
8. adularia (sulfate: feldspar group)
9. sunstone (sulfate: feldspar group)
10. fluorspar (fluorite)
11. amber (fossil resin)
12. coral
13. pearl
14. diamonds
15. not on this chart

ATTENTION: STONES, CRYSTALS, AND MINERALS ARE FOR
EXTERNAL USE ONLY!

LITERATURE ABOUT STONES, CRYSTALS, AND MINERALS PROVIDES
DETAILED INSIGHT INTO THEIR CORRECT APPLICATION.

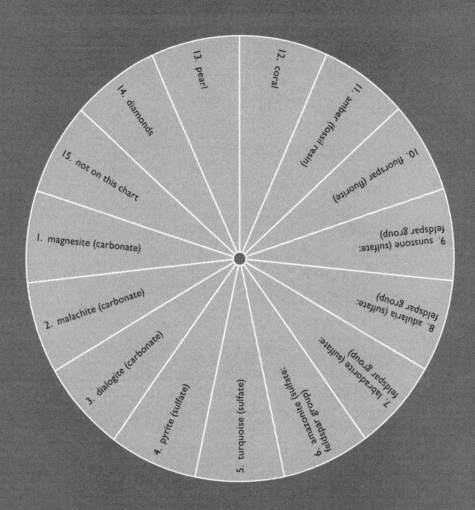

1. magnesite (carbonate)
2. malachite (carbonate)
3. dialogite (carbonate)
4. pyrite (sulfate)
5. turquoise (sulfate)
6. amazonite (sulfate: feldspar group)
7. labradorite (sulfate: feldspar group)
8. adularia (sulfate: feldspar group)
9. sunstone (sulfate: feldspar group)
10. fluorspar (fluorite)
11. amber (fossil resin)
12. coral
13. pearl
14. diamonds
15. not on this chart

Which stones, crystals, or minerals are of greatest use to me—#4?

CHART 54

Which metal is of greatest use to me?

1. aluminum
2. mercury
3. zinc
4. nickel
5. magnesium
6. antimony
7. pyrite
8. tin
9. copper
10. gold
11. lead
12. platinum
13. silver
14. iron
15. not on this chart

ATTENTION: METALS ARE FOR EXTERNAL USE ONLY!

LITERATURE ABOUT METALS PROVIDES DETAILED INSIGHT INTO THEIR CORRECT APPLICATION.

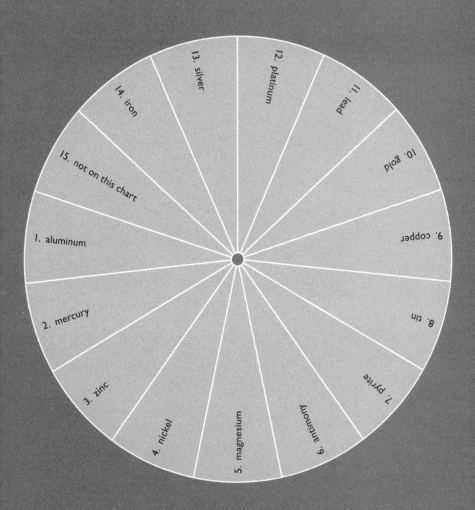

Which metal is of greatest use to me?

CHART 55

Which metal should I avoid?

1. aluminum
2. mercury
3. zinc
4. nickel
5. magnesium
6. antimony
7. pyrite
8. tin
9. copper
10. gold
11. lead
12. platinum
13. silver
14. iron
15. not on this chart

SEE ALSO PENDULUM CHARTS 12, 23, 24, 109, 119

ATTENTION: METALS ARE FOR EXTERNAL USE ONLY!

LITERATURE ABOUT METALS PROVIDES DETAILED INSIGHT INTO THEIR CORRECT APPLICATION.

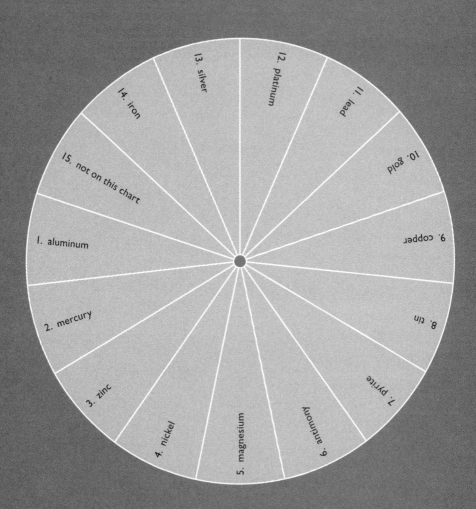

1. aluminum
2. mercury
3. zinc
4. nickel
5. magnesium
6. antimony
7. pyrite
8. tin
9. copper
10. gold
11. lead
12. platinum
13. silver
14. iron
15. not on this chart

Which metal should I avoid?

CHART 56

Which incense should I use—#1?

1. bergamot
2. myrrh
3. geranium
4. musk
5. lemongrass
6. sandalwood
7. vanilla
8. aloe
9. jasmine
10. copal
11. lavender
12. mandarin
13. cedar
14. benzoin
15. not on this chart

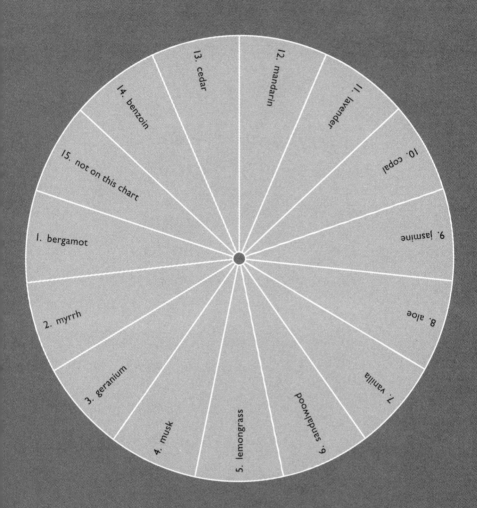

1. bergamot
2. myrrh
3. geranium
4. musk
5. lemongrass
6. sandalwood
7. vanilla
8. aloe
9. jasmine
10. copal
11. lavender
12. mandarin
13. cedar
14. benzoin
15. not on this chart

Which incense should I use—#1?

CHART 57

Which incense should I use—#2?

1. cypress
2. mastic
3. vetiver
4. olibanum (incense)
5. balsam incense
6. ylang-ylang
7. mimosa
8. patchouli
9. rose
10. costus root
11. pine
12. eucalyptus
13. galbanum
14. storax (amber)
15. not on this chart

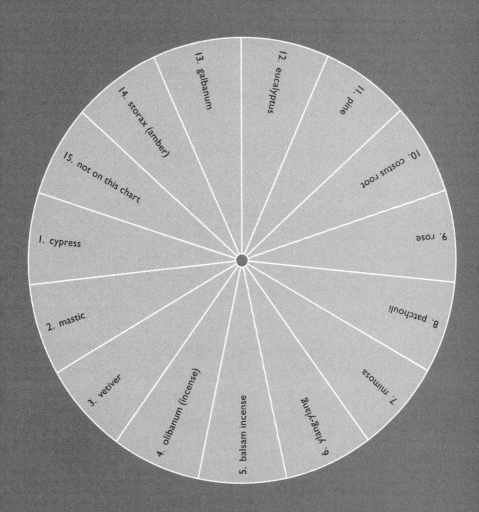

1. cypress
2. mastic
3. vetiver
4. olibanum (incense)
5. balsam incense
6. ylang-ylang
7. mimosa
8. patchouli
9. rose
10. costus root
11. pine
12. eucalyptus
13. galbanum
14. storax (amber)
15. not on this chart

Which incense should I use—#2?

CHART 58

Which bright color influences me in a positive way?

1. light yellow
2. dark yellow
3. light orange
4. dark orange
5. light red
6. dark red
7. light blue
8. dark blue
9. light violet
10. dark violet
11. light pink
12. dark pink
13. turquoise

14. light green
15. dark green
16. light brown
17. dark brown
18. light gray
19. dark gray
20. white (all colors)
21. black (no color)
22. silver
23. gold
24. no special color
25. not on this chart

LITERATURE ABOUT COLOR THERAPY PROVIDES DETAILED INSIGHT INTO THEIR PRECISE APPLICATION.

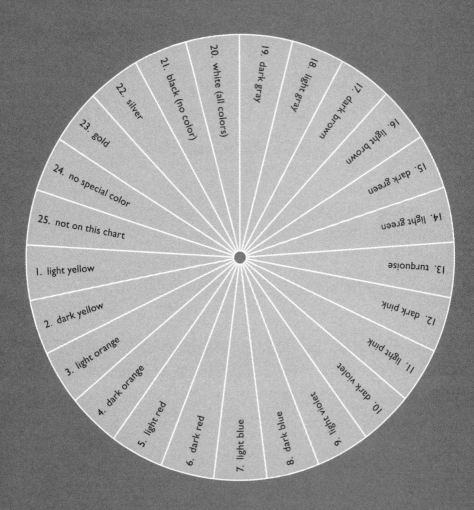

Which bright color influences me in a positive way?

22. silver
21. black (no color)
20. white (all colors)
19. dark gray
18. light gray
17. dark brown
16. light brown
15. dark green
14. light green
13. turquoise
12. dark pink
11. light pink
10. dark violet
9. light violet
8. dark blue
7. light blue
6. dark red
5. light red
4. dark orange
3. light orange
2. dark yellow
1. light yellow
25. not on this chart
24. no special color
23. gold

CHART 59

Which bright color should I avoid?

1. light yellow
2. dark yellow
3. light orange
4. dark orange
5. light red
6. dark red
7. light blue
8. dark blue
9. light violet
10. dark violet
11. light pink
12. dark pink
13. turquoise
14. light green
15. dark green
16. light brown
17. dark brown
18. light gray
19. dark gray
20. white (all colors)
21. black (no color)
22. silver
23. gold
24. no special color
25. not on this chart

LITERATURE ABOUT COLOR THERAPY PROVIDES DETAILED INSIGHT INTO THEIR PRECISE APPLICATION.

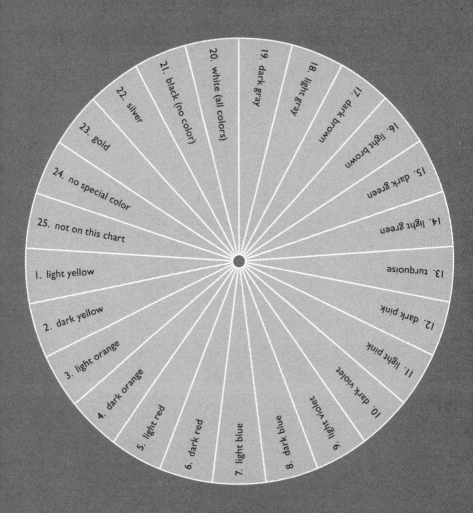

Which bright color should I avoid?

1. light yellow
2. dark yellow
3. light orange
4. dark orange
5. light red
6. dark red
7. light blue
8. dark blue
9. light violet
10. dark violet
11. light pink
12. dark pink
13. turquoise
14. light green
15. dark green
16. light brown
17. dark brown
18. light gray
19. dark gray
20. white (all colors)
21. black (no color)
22. silver
23. gold
24. no special color
25. not on this chart

CHART 60

Which pastel color influences me in a positive way?

1. pastel yellow
2. pastel orange
3. pastel red
4. pastel blue
5. pastel green
6. pastel pink
7. pastel violet
8. pastel turquoise
9. pastel brown
10. pastel gray
11. pastel white
12. sand colors
13. no special color
14. several colors
15. not on this chart

LITERATURE ABOUT COLOR THERAPY PROVIDES DETAILED INSIGHT INTO THEIR PRECISE APPLICATION.

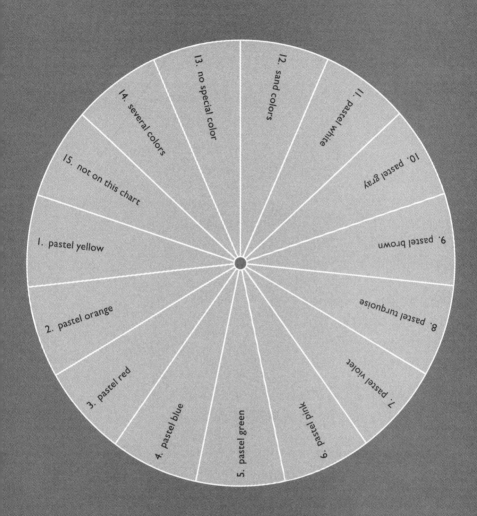

1. pastel yellow
2. pastel orange
3. pastel red
4. pastel blue
5. pastel green
6. pastel pink
7. pastel violet
8. pastel turquoise
9. pastel brown
10. pastel gray
11. pastel white
12. sand colors
13. no special color
14. several colors
15. not on this chart

Which pastel color influences me in a positive way?

CHART 61

Which pastel color should I avoid?

1. pastel yellow
2. pastel orange
3. pastel red
4. pastel blue
5. pastel green
6. pastel pink
7. pastel violet
8. pastel turquoise
9. pastel brown
10. pastel gray
11. pastel white
12. sand colors
13. no special color
14. several colors
15. not on this chart

LITERATURE ABOUT COLOR THERAPY PROVIDES DETAILED INSIGHT INTO THEIR PRECISE APPLICATION.

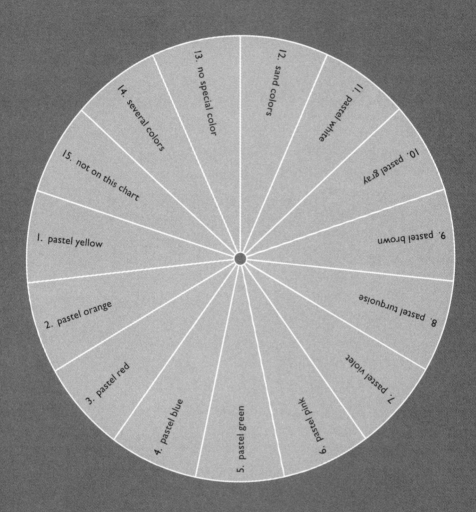

Which pastel color should I avoid?

CHART 62

What form of meditation suits me best?

1. vipassana meditation
2. visual meditation
3. energetic meditation
4. mantra meditation
5. kundalini meditation
6. chakra meditation
7. color meditation
8. crystal meditation
9. respiratory meditation
10. sun meditation
11. mandala meditation
12. Christian meditation
13. Buddhist meditation
14. Zen meditation
15. not on this chart

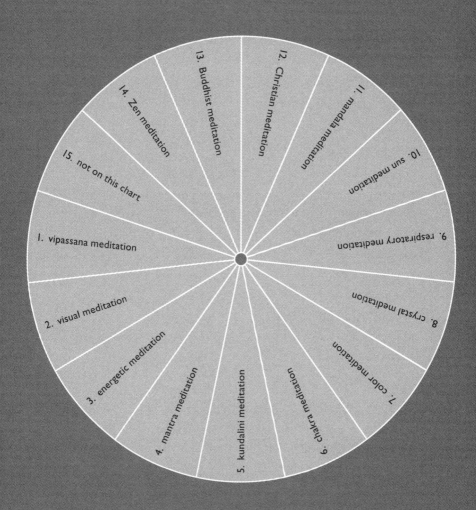

1. vipassana meditation
2. visual meditation
3. energetic meditation
4. mantra meditation
5. kundalini meditation
6. chakra meditation
7. color meditation
8. crystal meditation
9. respiratory meditation
10. sun meditation
11. mandala meditation
12. Christian meditation
13. Buddhist meditation
14. Zen meditation
15. not on this chart

What form of meditation suits me best?

CHART 63

What alternative medical treatment will work best for me?

1. reiki
2. homeopathy
3. light therapy
4. sound therapy
5. color therapy
6. aromatherapy
7. Bach flower therapy
8. neurolinguistic programming (NLP)
9. herbal therapy
10. acupuncture
11. chakra work
12. meditation therapy
13. body work (massage, etc.)
14. precious stone therapy
15. not on this chart

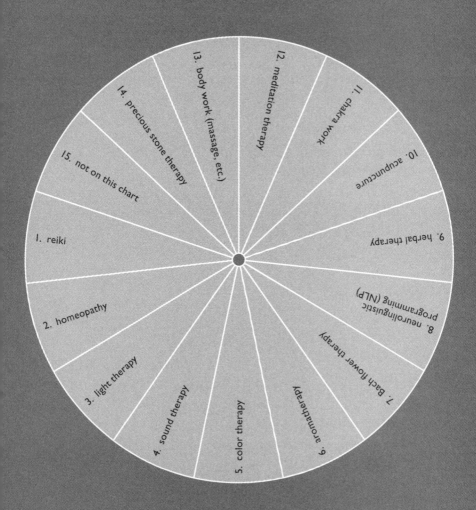

1. reiki
2. homeopathy
3. light therapy
4. sound therapy
5. color therapy
6. aromatherapy
7. Bach flower therapy
8. neurolinguistic programming (NLP)
9. herbal therapy
10. acupuncture
11. chakra work
12. meditation therapy
13. body work (massage, etc.)
14. precious stone therapy
15. not on this chart

What alternative medical treatment will work best for me?

CHART 64

Which therapy or medical treatment will give me the most vitality?

1. qui gong
2. bioenergetics
3. shiatsu
4. Chinese medicine
5. respiratory therapy
6. energetic meditation
7. reiki
8. tai chi
9. laying on of hands
10. chakra work
11. magnet therapy
12. homeopathy
13. hypnosis
14. visual mediation
15. rebalancing energy
16. rebirthing
17. yoga
18. overtone singing
19. Reichian therapy
20. fasting
21. autogenic training
22. acupuncture
23. kinesiology
24. breathwork
25. not on this chart

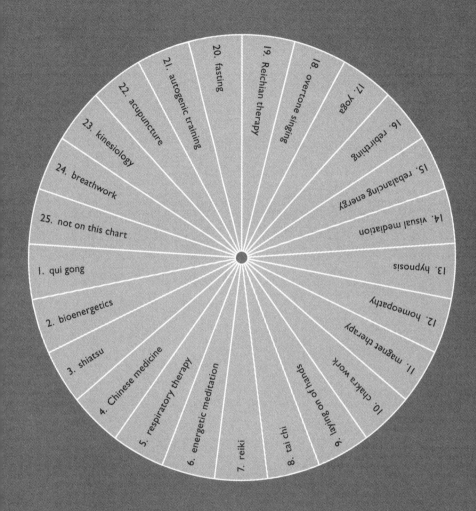

1. qui gong
2. bioenergetics
3. shiatsu
4. Chinese medicine
5. respiratory therapy
6. energetic meditation
7. reiki
8. tai chi
9. laying on of hands
10. chakra work
11. magnet therapy
12. homeopathy
13. hypnosis
14. visual meditation
15. rebalancing energy
16. rebirthing
17. yoga
18. overtone singing
19. Reichian therapy
20. fasting
21. autogenic training
22. acupuncture
23. kinesiology
24. breathwork
25. not on this chart

Which therapy or medical treatment will give me the most vitality?

CHART 65

What unconscious issues are determining my life?

1. control
2. emotional security
3. fear
4. fulfillment
5. creativity
6. perception
7. understanding
8. freedom
9. spontaneity
10. financial profit
11. recognition
12. self-interest
13. self-esteem
14. obedience
15. not on this chart

SEE ALSO PENDULUM CHARTS 36, 66 TO 71

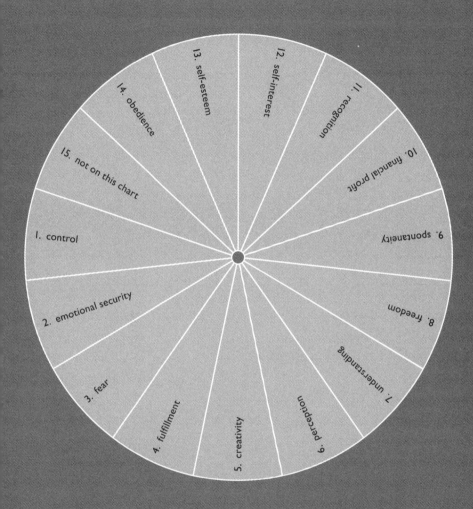

What unconscious issues are determining my life?

1. control
2. emotional security
3. fear
4. fulfillment
5. creativity
6. perception
7. understanding
8. freedom
9. spontaneity
10. financial profit
11. recognition
12. self-interest
13. self-esteem
14. obedience
15. not on this chart

CHART 66

Which guiding principle is particularly important to me today?

1. initiative
2. inspiration
3. compassion
4. friendship
5. collaboration
6. success
7. understanding
8. perspective
9. balance
10. humor
11. spirituality
12. love
13. perseverance
14. self-esteem
15. not on this chart

SEE ALSO PENDULUM CHARTS 36, 65, 67 TO 71

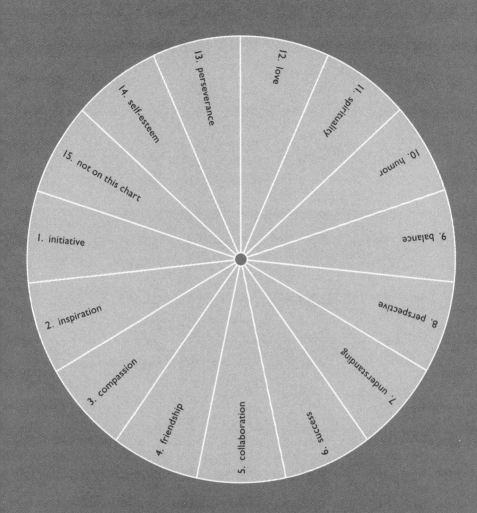

Which guiding principle is particularly important to me today?

CHART 67

What matter/s should I concentrate on—particularly today?

1. confiding in someone
2. new ideas
3. an important encounter
4. an important event
5. cleaning up
6. taking a chance
7. taking up a forgotten plan
8. realizing a long held desire
9. carrying out good resolution
10. putting aside "hopeless" things
11. following the path set upon
12. having confidence in a happy ending
13. going through matters in proper order
14. recognizing my deepest feelings
15. not on this chart

SEE ALSO PENDULUM CHARTS 36, 65, 66, 68 TO 71

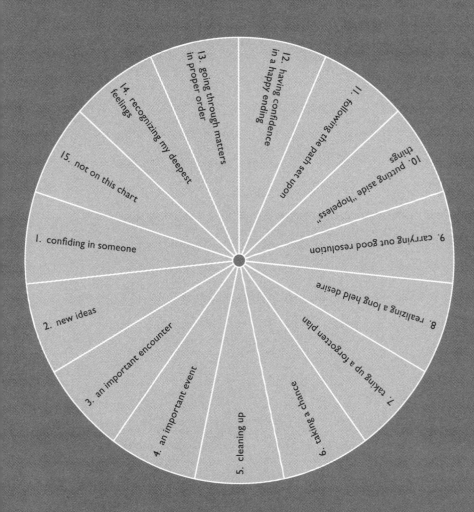

1. confiding in someone
2. new ideas
3. an important encounter
4. an important event
5. cleaning up
6. taking a chance
7. taking up a forgotten plan
8. realizing a long held desire
9. carrying out good resolution
10. putting aside "hopeless" things
11. following the path set upon
12. having confidence in a happy ending
13. going through matters in proper order
14. recognizing my deepest feelings
15. not on this chart

What matter/s should I concentrate on—particularly today?

CHART 68

How can I make changes in the most important things in my life?

1. set energy free
2. believe firmly in them
3. keep eyes and ears open
4. become proactive
5. keep the goal in sight
6. create order
7. look from a different perspective
8. work on them
9. hang in there
10. forgive myself
11. take the chance
12. release myself from a burden
13. seek help from others
14. listen to myself
15. not on this chart

SEE ALSO PENDULUM CHARTS 36, 65 TO 67, 69 TO 71

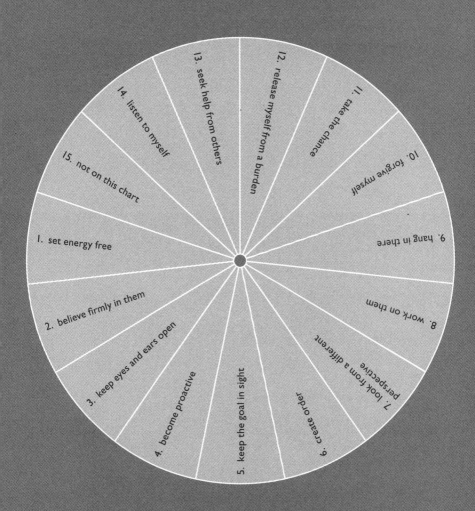

13. seek help from others
12. release myself from a burden
14. listen to myself
11. take the chance
15. not on this chart
10. forgive myself
1. set energy free
9. hang in there
2. believe firmly in them
8. work on them
3. keep eyes and ears open
7. look from a different perspective
4. become proactive
6. create order
5. keep the goal in sight

How can I make changes in the most important things in my life?

CHART 69

What is preventing me from reaching my goal?

1. disappointment
2. rage
3. bitterness
4. no confidence
5. boredom
6. confusion
7. denial
8. desperation
9. dishonesty
10. doubt
11. jealousy
12. fear
13. feelings of guilt
14. prejudice
15. grief
16. greed
17. fear of being abandoned
18. a leaning toward escape
19. too much criticism
20. fear of failing
21. mistrust
22. avarice
23. irresponsibility
24. moodiness
25. not on this chart

SEE ALSO PENDULUM CHARTS 36, 65 TO 68, 70, 71

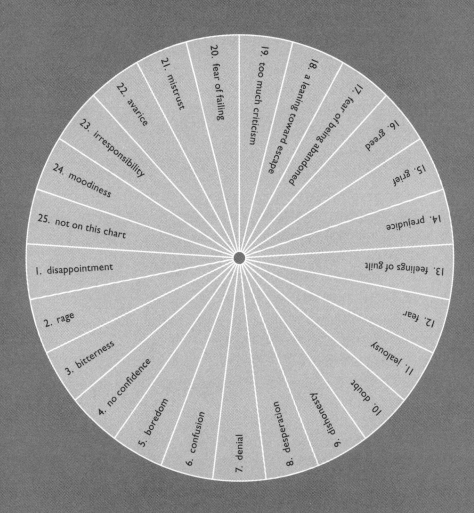

1. disappointment
2. rage
3. bitterness
4. no confidence
5. boredom
6. confusion
7. denial
8. desperation
9. dishonesty
10. doubt
11. jealousy
12. fear
13. feelings of guilt
14. prejudice
15. grief
16. greed
17. fear of being abandoned
18. a leaning toward escape
19. too much criticism
20. fear of failing
21. mistrust
22. avarice
23. irresponsibility
24. moodiness
25. not on this chart

What is preventing me from reaching my goal?

CHART 70

Which statement impedes my inner growth and spirituality?

1. I will never succeed in this
2. I receive too little recognition
3. I will never learn this
4. I am not suited for this
5. I have no chance
6. I can't do this alone
7. I cannot influence this situation
8. I never get a real chance
9. I am not taken seriously
10. someone is begrudging something
11. I know exactly what I am doing
12. I do not need help from anyone
13. I can stand my ground
14. I know what others are thinking
15. I have everything under control
16. I can't do anything about it anyhow
17. I would never dare
18. I can't confide in anyone
19. I owe it to him/her
20. I owe it to myself
21. it doesn't matter to me
22. I am indebted to him/her/it
23. I can always come back to it later
24. criticism doesn't matter to me
25. not on this chart

SEE ALSO PENDULUM CHARTS 36, 65 TO 69, 71

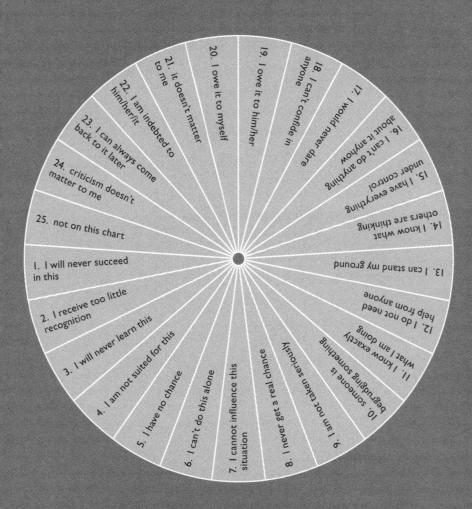

Which statement impedes my inner growth and spirituality?

The wheel segments read (clockwise from top):

20. I owe it to myself
19. I owe it to him/her
18. I can't confide in anyone
17. I would never dare
16. I can't do anything about it anyhow
15. I have everything under control
14. I know what others are thinking
13. I can stand my ground
12. I do not need help from anyone
11. I know exactly what I am doing
10. someone is begrudging something
9. I am not taken seriously
8. I never get a real chance
7. I cannot influence this situation
6. I can't do this alone
5. I have no chance
4. I am not suited for this
3. I will never learn this
2. I receive too little recognition
1. I will never succeed in this
25. not on this chart
24. criticism doesn't matter to me
23. I can always come back to it later
22. I am indebted to him/her/it
21. it doesn't matter to me

CHART 71

What do I need to take into account in my everyday life?

1. I occupy myself with pleasant things
2. I dare to create my own atmosphere
3. I surround myself with nice people
4. that I let things run their course
5. that I see my friends regularly
6. that I take enough time for my hobby
7. that I don't live in a fantasy world
8. I burden myself with too many things
9. that I not worry too much
10. that I need to go wild once in a while
11. that I let myself be carried away
12. that I plan too much
13. that I have fun
14. that I enjoy the moment
15. not on this chart

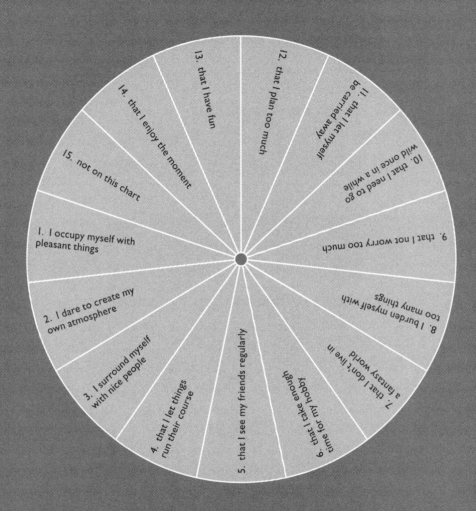

What do I need to take into account in my everyday life?

1. I occupy myself with pleasant things
2. I dare to create my own atmosphere
3. I surround myself with nice people
4. that I let things run their course
5. that I see my friends regularly
6. that I take enough time for my hobby
7. that I don't live in a fantasy world
8. I burden myself with too many things
9. that I not worry too much
10. that I need to go wild once in a while
11. that I let myself be carried away
12. that I plan too much
13. that I have fun
14. that I enjoy the moment
15. not on this chart

CHART 72

Developing my spirituality is important to me because:

1. it offers me the possibility of growing
2. it gives me what I otherwise lack
3. it offers me a way to communicate
4. it offers me a way to accept myself as I am
5. it offers me a way to accept others as they are
6. it has revealed dimensions of life
7. I remain curious about the unknown
8. I can be open to other human beings
9. I can overcome my limitations
10. I have gotten to know my desires
11. each day I learn something new
12. it offers freedom to "color" my life
13. everything has a meaning
14. I dare to trust in the unknown
15. not on this chart

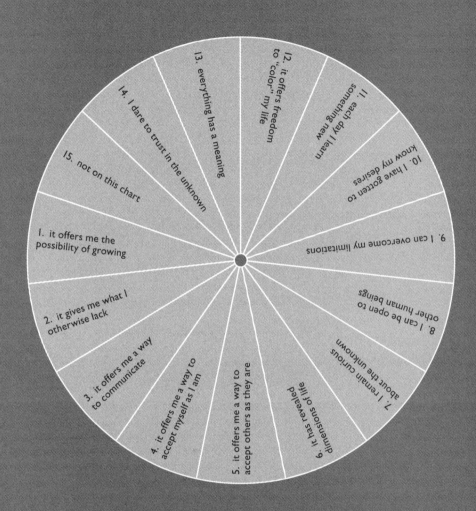

1. it offers me the possibility of growing
2. it gives me what I otherwise lack
3. it offers me a way to communicate
4. it offers me a way to accept myself as I am
5. it offers me a way to accept others as they are
6. it has revealed dimensions of life
7. I remain curious about the unknown
8. I can be open to other human beings
9. I can overcome my limitations
10. I have gotten to know my desires
11. each day I learn something new
12. it offers freedom to "color" my life
13. everything has a meaning
14. I dare to trust in the unknown
15. not on this chart

Developing my spirituality is important to me because:

CHART 73

I gain inspiration from _____.

1. the atmosphere I create
2. the people in my immediate surrounding
3. nature
4. meditation
5. love
6. traveling
7. solitude
8. my dreams
9. my friends
10. my family
11. my belief in myself
12. risk-taking
13. my work
14. gratitude
15. not on this chart

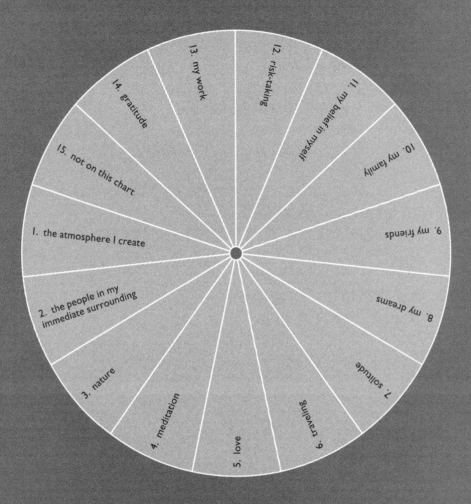

13. my work

12. risk-taking

14. gratitude

11. my belief in myself

15. not on this chart

10. my family

1. the atmosphere I create

9. my friends

2. the people in my immediate surrounding

8. my dreams

3. nature

7. solitude

4. meditation

6. traveling

5. love

I gain inspiration from _____.

CHART 74

*Ambition is important to me because*_____.

1. it offers me satisfaction
2. it inspires me
3. I feel a responsibility to use my talent
4. I want to succeed in life
5. I like to hold an important position
6. I can put my energy into it
7. I want my achievements to be better
8. I can live my creativity through it
9. I want to realize my plans for the future
10. I like to be in the limelight
11. I want to grow at all times
12. I want to show what I can do
13. I am curious about new things
14. I can bear a lot of responsibility
15. not on this chart

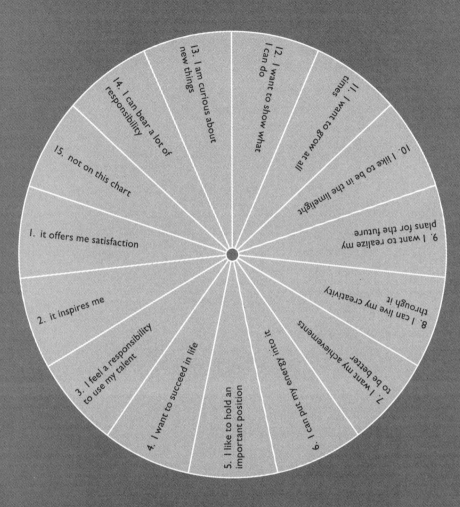

14. I can bear a lot of responsibility

13. I am curious about new things

12. I want to show what I can do

11. I want to grow at all times

10. I like to be in the limelight

9. I want to realize my plans for the future

8. I can live my creativity through it

7. I want my achievements to be better

6. I can put my energy into it

5. I like to hold an important position

4. I want to succeed in life

3. I feel a responsibility to use my talent

2. it inspires me

1. it offers me satisfaction

15. not on this chart

Ambition is important to me because _____.

CHART 75

To me, success means _____.

1. confidence in my skills
2. recognition for my work
3. personal growth
4. collaboration
5. new possibilities
6. satisfaction
7. making progress
8. development
9. joy
10. never standing still
11. an essential part of my life
12. confidence in others
13. relaxation
14. stable relationships
15. not on this chart

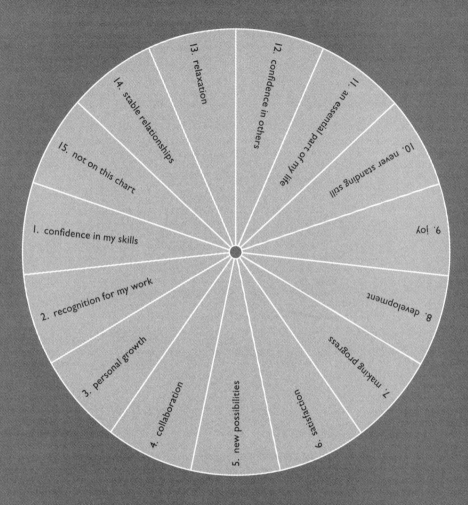

To me, success means _____.

CHART 76

Who plays a very significant role in my life?

1. father
2. mother
3. younger brother(s)
4. younger sister(s)
5. older brother(s)
6. older sister(s)
7. partner/relationship
8. child(ren)
9. teacher/instructor
10. colleague(s)
11. reliable person
12. best friend/best buddy
13. I myself
14. employer
15. fellow student
16. neighbor
17. pen friend
18. close relative(s)
19. circle of friends
20. someone I know through my job
21. someone I know through my hobby
22. distant relatives
23. a new acquaintance
24. an old friend/acquaintance
25. not on this chart

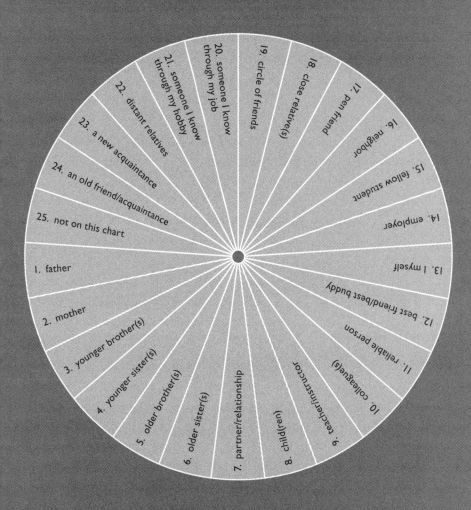

1. father
2. mother
3. younger brother(s)
4. younger sister(s)
5. older brother(s)
6. older sister(s)
7. partner/relationship
8. child(ren)
9. teacher/instructor
10. colleague(s)
11. reliable person
12. best friend/best buddy
13. I myself
14. employer
15. fellow student
16. neighbor
17. pen friend
18. close relative(s)
19. circle of friends
20. someone I know through my job
21. someone I know through my hobby
22. distant relatives
23. a new acquaintance
24. an old friend/acquaintance
25. not on this chart

Who plays a very significant role in my life?

CHART 77

Which oracle or guiding principle will work best for me?

1. Tarot
2. I Ching
3. runes
4. numerology
5. astrology
6. pendulum work
7. psychic readings
8. geomancy
9. laying out cards
10. meditation
11. power cards
12. oracle cards
13. my intuition
14. channeling
15. not on this chart

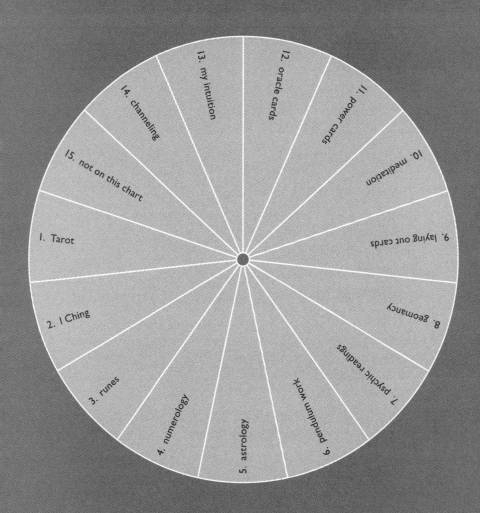

14. channeling
13. my intuition
12. oracle cards
11. power cards
10. meditation
9. laying out cards
8. geomancy
7. psychic readings
6. pendulum work
5. astrology
4. numerology
3. runes
2. I Ching
1. Tarot
15. not on this chart

Which oracle or guiding principle will work best for me?

CHART 78

Which Tarot card is most meaningful to me today?

1. The Magician
2. The High Priestess
3. The Empress
4. The Emperor
5. The Hierophant
6. The Lovers
7. The Chariot
8. Strength
9. The Hermit
10. The Wheel of Fortune
11. Justice
12. The Hanged Man
13. Death
14. Temperance
15. The Devil
16. The Tower
17. The Star
18. The Moon
19. The Sun
20. Judgment
21. The World
22. The Fool
23. several possibilities
24. no certain card
25. not on this chart

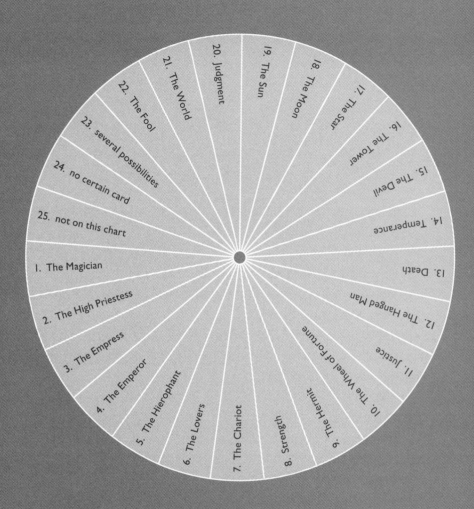

Which Tarot card is most meaningful to me today?

CHART 79

Which rune is most meaningful to me today?

1. Fehu
2. Uruz
3. Thurisaz
4. Ansuz
5. Raidho
6. Kenaz
7. Gebo
8. Wunjo
9. Hagalaz
10. Naudhiz
11. Isa
12. Jera
13. Eihwaz
14. Perdhro
15. Algiz
16. Sowulo
17. Tiwaz
18. Berkana
19. Eihwaz
20. Mannaz
21. Laguz
22. Ingwaz
23. Dagaz
24. Othala
25. not on this chart

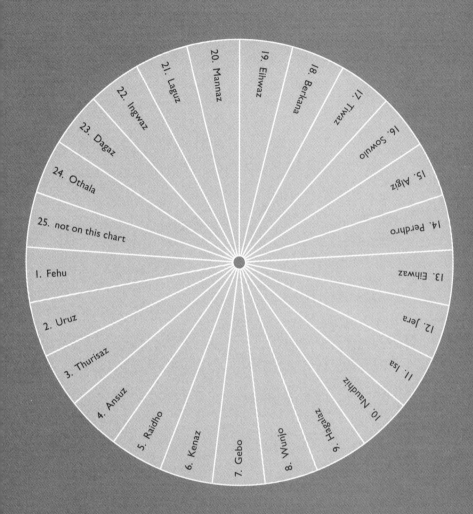

Which rune is most meaningful to me today?

CHART 80

What is my ascendant?

1. Aries
2. Taurus
3. Gemini
4. Cancer
5. Leo
6. Virgo
7. Libra
8. Scorpio
9. Sagittarius
10. Capricorn
11. Aquarius
12. Pisces
13. there is too little information ...
14. no choice possible
15. not on this chart

USE THIS CHART ONLY IF THE PRECISE INFORMATION REGARDING THE HOUR OF YOUR BIRTH IS MISSING!

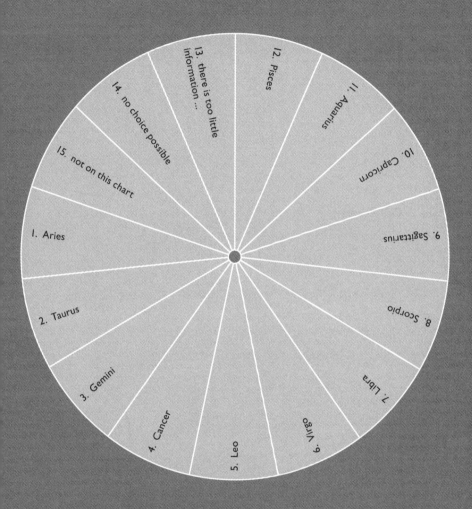

What is my ascendant?

CHART 81

Which planet and/or which element influences me most of all?

1. Sun
2. Moon
3. Mercury
4. Venus
5. Mars
6. Jupiter
7. Saturn
8. Uranus
9. Neptune
10. Pluto
11. fire
12. earth
13. air
14. water
15. not on this chart

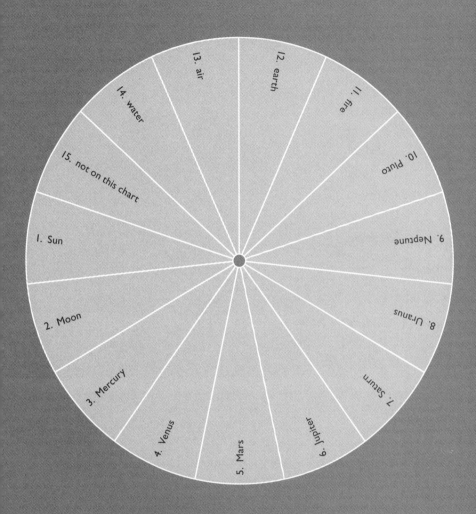

Which planet and/or which element influences me most of all?

CHART 82

Which house has the greatest influence on me today?

1. House 1
2. House 2
3. House 3
4. House 4
5. House 5
6. House 6
7. House 7
8. House 8
9. House 9
10. House 10
11. House 11
12. House 12
13. several possibilities
14. no choice possible
15. not on this chart

USE THIS CHART ONLY IF THE PRECISE INFORMATION REGARDING THE HOUR OF YOUR BIRTH IS MISSING!

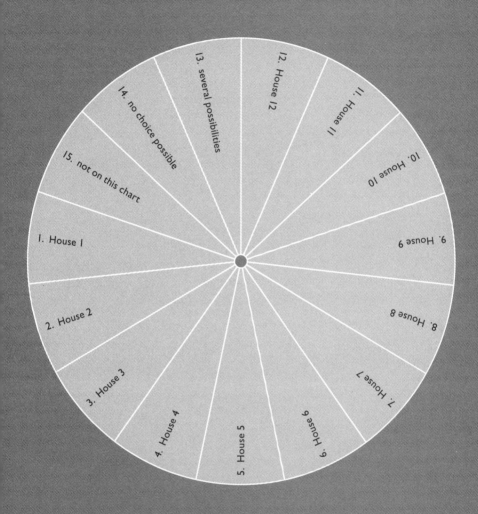

Which house has the greatest influence on me today?

CHART 83

What characteristic describes me best?

1. enthusiastic
2. playful
3. gullible
4. persevering
5. serious
6. philosophical
7. practical
8. energetic
9. curious
10. eager to learn
11. dreamy
12. generous
13. warm
14. conservative
15. cautious
16. sensitive
17. sensible
18. good intellectual grasp
19. sympathetic
20. passionate
21. stable
22. emotional
23. sensual
24. strong
25. not on this chart

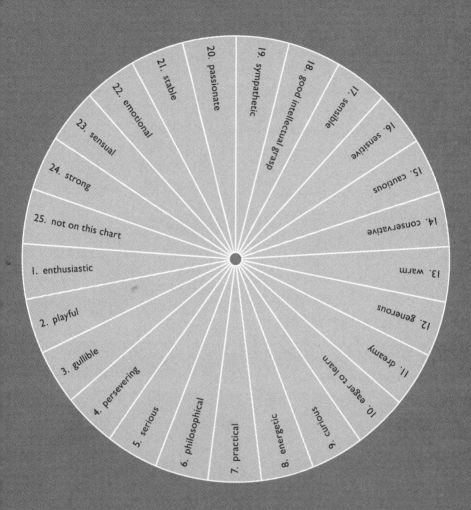

What characteristic describes me best?

20. passionate
21. stable
22. emotional
23. sensual
24. strong
25. not on this chart
1. enthusiastic
2. playful
3. gullible
4. persevering
5. serious
6. philosophical
7. practical
8. energetic
9. curious
10. eager to learn
11. dreamy
12. generous
13. warm
14. conservative
15. cautious
16. sensitive
17. sensible
18. good intellectual grasp
19. sympathetic

CHART 84

Which statement describes me best, according to others?

1. I wear myself out chasing after things
2. I see which way the wind is blowing
3. slow but sure wins the race
4. where there's a will, there's a way
5. problems are there to be solved
6. I don't dwell on my mistakes
7. there's a good side to everything
8. when life shuts the door . . .
9. I keep my head up
10. a good start is half the battle
11. time will bring an answer
12. money is for spending
13. if i don't do it nobody will
14. friendship means everything to me
15. "quitting" not in my vocabulary
16. waste not, want not
17. I don't give anything away
18. fun forever
19. I don't live for work
20. my house is your house
21. you have to get up pretty early . . .
22. a good start is half the work
23. mistakes are there to learn from
24. sunshine follows the rain
25. not on this chart

SEE ALSO PENDULUM CHARTS 83, 93, 94

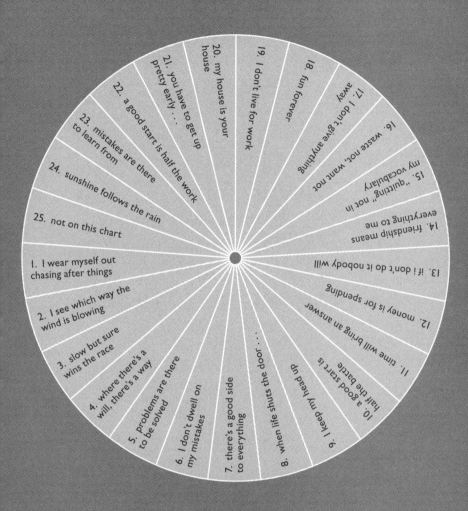

Which statement describes me best, according to others?

1. I wear myself out chasing after things
2. I see which way the wind is blowing
3. slow but sure wins the race
4. where there's a will, there's a way
5. problems are there to be solved
6. I don't dwell on my mistakes
7. there's a good side to everything
8. when life shuts the door . . . .
9. I keep my head up
10. a good start is half the battle
11. time will bring an answer
12. money is for spending
13. if I don't do it nobody will
14. friendship means everything to me
15. "quitting" not in my vocabulary
16. waste not, want not
17. I don't give anything away
18. fun forever
19. I don't live for work
20. my house is your house
21. you have to get up pretty early . . .
22. a good start is half the work
23. mistakes are there to learn from
24. sunshine follows the rain
25. not on this chart

CHART 85

Which statement describes my social life?

1. I like to be among people
2. I am easy to get along with
3. I am always the life of the party
4. I can talk to anyone
5. I can calm people
6. I am obliging and polite
7. I want to please everybody
8. people really interest me
9. I nurture my friendships
10. I have a great sense of humor
11. I hear news through the grapevine
12. I like to be the focus of attention
13. I'm a good listener
14. I know how to enchant people
15. I never gossip about my friends
16. I like to help others
17. I am almost never alone
18. I like to interfere with other people
19. I'd rather not go to a party alone
20. I am often late
21. I often forget about meetings
22. I can't find anything to talk about . . .
23. I don't like to being in groups
24. I would rather be alone
25. not on this chart

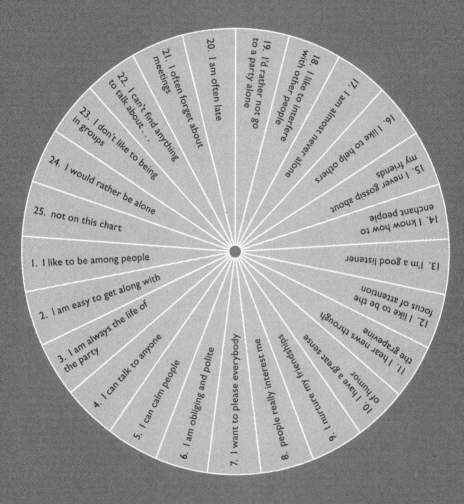

1. I like to be among people
2. I am easy to get along with
3. I am always the life of the party
4. I can talk to anyone
5. I can calm people
6. I am obliging and polite
7. I want to please everybody
8. people really interest me
9. I nurture my friendships
10. I have a great sense of humor
11. I hear news through the grapevine
12. I like to be the focus of attention
13. I'm a good listener
14. I know how to enchant people
15. I never gossip about my friends
16. I like to help others
17. I am almost never alone
18. I like to interfere with other people
19. I'd rather not go to a party alone
20. I am often late
21. I often forget about meetings
22. I can't find anything to talk about...
23. I don't like to being in groups
24. I would rather be alone
25. not on this chart

Which statement describes my social life?

CHART 86

Which statement describes my professional life?

1. I have a great sense of responsibility
2. I like to manage things for others
3. I know how to call attention . . .
4. I take too much responsibility . . .
5. I am too chaotic
6. I am a good team player
7. I don't let myself be influenced by gossip
8. I generally help my colleagues
9. I give others the feeling . . .
10. I try to become closer to colleagues
11. I try to become closer to my boss
12. I often push responsibility off . . .
13. I entrench myself behind my work
14. I see to it that I always look neat
15. I am never late
16. I never complain about boring tasks
17. I try to get out of boring work-tasks
18. I try to make a good impression . . .
19. I cannot identify with my work
20. I can identify well with my work
21. I feel comfortable as part of a team
22. I prefer working alone
23. I react enthusiastically to new . . .
24. I can estimate my personal potential . . .
25. not on this chart

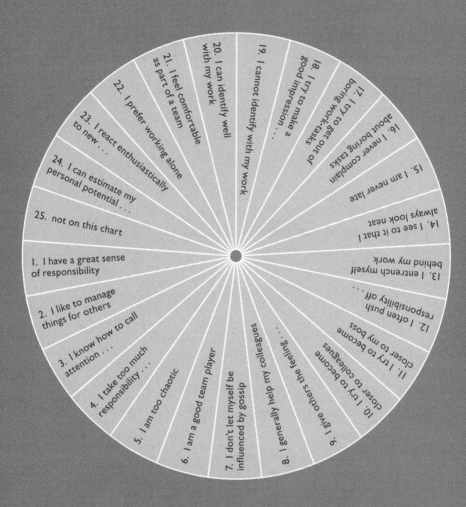

20. I can identify well with my work
21. I feel comfortable as part of a team
22. I prefer working alone
23. I react enthusiastically to new . . .
24. I can estimate my personal potential . . .
25. not on this chart
1. I have a great sense of responsibility
2. I like to manage things for others
3. I know how to call attention . . .
4. I take too much responsibility . . .
5. I am too chaotic
6. I am a good team player
7. I don't let myself be influenced by gossip
8. I generally help my colleagues
9. I give others the feeling . . .
10. I try to become closer to colleagues
11. I try to become closer to my boss
12. I often push responsibility off . . .
13. I entrench myself behind my work
14. I see to it that I always look neat
15. I am never late
16. I never complain about boring tasks
17. I try to get out of boring work-tasks
18. I try to make a good impression . . .
19. I cannot identify with my work

Which statement describes my professional life?

CHART 87

My personality corresponds to what enneagram type—#1?

1. I make decisions quickly and safely
2. I am a perfectionist
3. I am impatient
4. I tend to criticize and moralize
5. I am afraid of being poor when old
6. I always make a lot of plans
7. my affairs are carefully arranged
8. I am good at saving
9. I am practical and energetic
10. I reach my goal by assisting others
11. I have inferiority complexes
12. I am vain
13. I demand recognition
14. I tend to be manipulative
15. I am very social
16. I complain easily
17. my career comes first
18. I am disciplined
19. I am afraid to fail
20. I attach importance to my image
21. I play a role . . .
22. I tend to be a workaholic
23. I do not show my feelings . . .
24. I manipulate people and situations
25. not on this chart

THIS CHART OFFERS SEVERAL POSSIBLE ANSWERS.

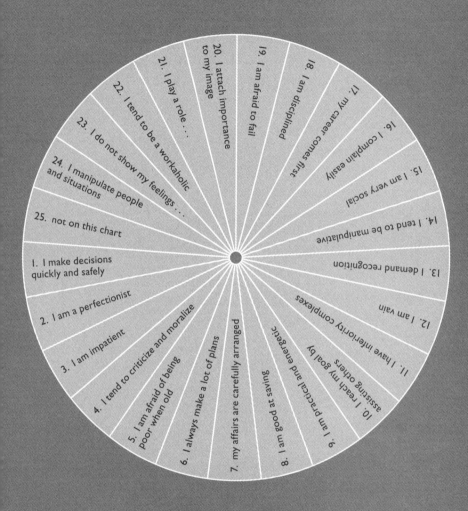

20. I attach importance to my image
21. I play a role . . .
22. I tend to be a workaholic
23. I do not show my feelings . . .
24. I manipulate people and situations
25. not on this chart
1. I make decisions quickly and safely
2. I am a perfectionist
3. I am impatient
4. I tend to criticize and moralize
5. I am afraid of being poor when old
6. I always make a lot of plans
7. my affairs are carefully arranged
8. I am good at saving
9. I am practical and energetic
10. I reach my goal by assisting others
11. I have inferiority complexes
12. I am vain
13. I demand recognition
14. I tend to be manipulative
15. I am very social
16. I complain easily
17. my career comes first
18. I am disciplined
19. I am afraid to fail

My personality corresponds to what enneagram type—#1?

CHART 88

My personality corresponds to what enneagram type—#2?

1. I am very creative
2. I am moody and unpredictable
3. I am envious
4. I am hypersensitive
5. I am very reserved
6. I feel special and "different" . . .
7. I can become very emotional
8. I tend to be a melancholic
9. I have a strong urge for knowledge
10. I quickly draw back . . .
11. I am distrustful
12. I am afraid of my feelings
13. although I know a lot . . .
14. I am optimistic
15. I hide behind my intellectual image
16. I am patient
17. I don't like to decide things alone
18. I am uncertain
19. I am very loyal
20. I have a sense of duty
21. I am persevering and determined
22. during conflicts I can stay calm . . .
23. I am capable of assessing my . . .
24. I like standing behind a higher . . .
25. not on this chart

THIS CHART OFFERS SEVERAL POSSIBLE ANSWERS.

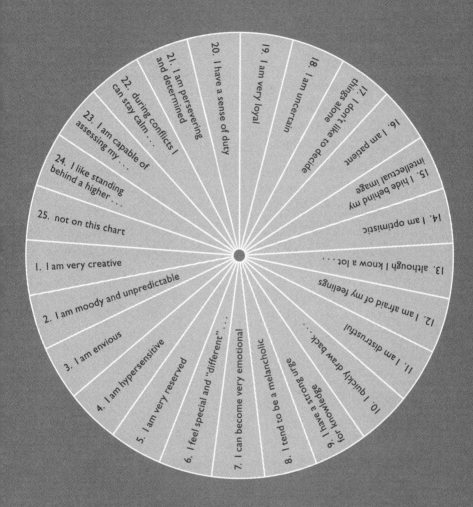

The wheel contains the following numbered segments:

1. I am very creative
2. I am moody and unpredictable
3. I am envious
4. I am hypersensitive
5. I am very reserved
6. I feel special and "different"...
7. I can become very emotional
8. I tend to be a melancholic
9. I have a strong urge for knowledge
10. I quickly draw back...
11. I am distrustful...
12. I am afraid of my feelings
13. although I know a lot...
14. I am optimistic
15. I hide behind my intellectual image
16. I am patient
17. I don't like to decide things alone
18. I am uncertain
19. I am very loyal
20. I have a sense of duty
21. I am persevering and determined
22. during conflicts I can stay calm...
23. I am capable of assessing my...
24. I like standing behind a higher...
25. not on this chart

My personality corresponds to what enneagram type—#2?

CHART 89

My personality corresponds to what enneagram type—#3?

1. I have quick powers . . .
2. I work on several things . . .
3. I am very optimistic
4. I radiate a childlike . . .
5. social contact is easy for me
6. I want to have as much fun . . .
7. I am interested in many . . .
8. I am a "lucky devil"
9. I have great self-confidence
10. I can weigh situations . . .
11. I protect the underdog
12. I can easily twist a situation . . .
13. I have a lot of staying power
14. I tend to use others . . .
15. I tend to control others . . .
16. I have a distinct sense . . .
17. I am passive . . .
18. I am gentle
19. I first become active . . .
20. I prefer to avoid conflicts
21. I appreciate my peace . . .
22. I am good with . . .
23. I strive for a harmonious . . .
24. I put other people's needs . . .
25. not on this chart

THIS CHART OFFERS SEVERAL POSSIBLE ANSWERS.

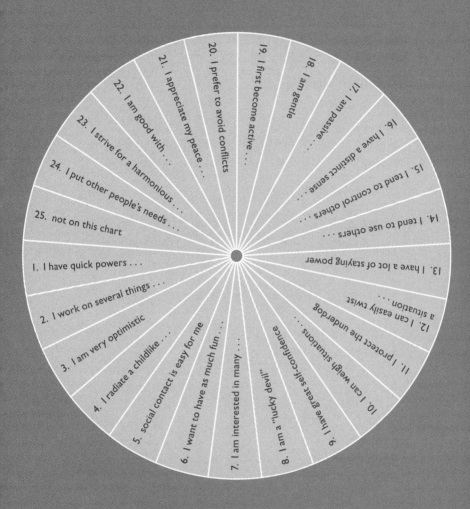

1. I have quick powers . . .
2. I work on several things . . .
3. I am very optimistic
4. I radiate a childlike . . .
5. social contact is easy for me
6. I want to have as much fun . . .
7. I am interested in many . . .
8. I am a "lucky devil"
9. I have great self-confidence . . .
10. I can weigh situations . . .
11. I protect the underdog
12. I can easily twist a situation . . .
13. I have a lot of staying power
14. I tend to use others . . .
15. I tend to control others . . .
16. I have a distinct sense . . .
17. I am passive . . .
18. I am gentle
19. I first become active . . .
20. I prefer to avoid conflicts
21. I appreciate my peace . . .
22. I am good with . . .
23. I strive for a harmonious . . .
24. I put other people's needs . . .
25. not on this chart

My personality corresponds to what enneagram type—#3?

CHART 90

What further training will have the most positive effect on my education/profession/talent?

1. administration
2. secretarial
3. public relations
4. trade
5. accounting
6. one or more languages
7. graphics
8. computer
9. management
10. law
11. economics
12. business administration
13. teaching elementary school
14. professor
15. therapy
16. veterinary medicine
17. alternative medicine
18. journalism/editorial
19. health care
20. bodywork techniques
21. beautician/hairstylist, etc.
22. ballet/dance
23. music
24. physical/sport
25. not on this chart

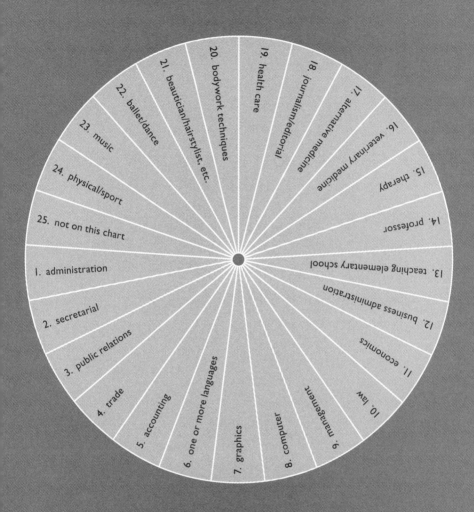

What further training will have the most positive effect on my education/profession/talent?

The wheel contains the following numbered segments:

1. administration
2. secretarial
3. public relations
4. trade
5. accounting
6. one or more languages
7. graphics
8. computer
9. management
10. law
11. economics
12. business administration
13. teaching elementary school
14. professor
15. therapy
16. veterinary medicine
17. alternative medicine
18. journalism/editorial
19. health care
20. bodywork techniques
21. beautician/hairstylist, etc.
22. ballet/dance
23. music
24. physical/sport
25. not on this chart

CHART 91

Which professional area suits me well?

1. art
2. teaching
3. craftsmanship
4. business
5. service industry
6. health care
7. bodywork techniques
8. agriculture
9. forestry
10. sales
11. banking/stock market
12. communications
13. law
14. medicine
15. architecture
16. management and organization
17. electronics and computer
18. advertising
19. government
20. politics
21. physical therapy/sports
22. hotel and gastronomy
23. media and journalism
24. engineer/designer/inventor
25. not on this chart

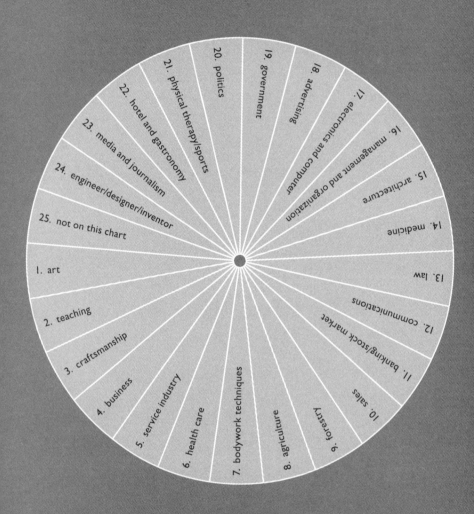

Which professional area suits me well?

1. art
2. teaching
3. craftsmanship
4. business
5. service industry
6. health care
7. bodywork techniques
8. agriculture
9. forestry
10. sales
11. banking/stock market
12. communications
13. law
14. medicine
15. architecture
16. management and organization
17. electronics and computer
18. advertising
19. government
20. politics
21. physical therapy/sports
22. hotel and gastronomy
23. media and journalism
24. engineer/designer/inventor
25. not on this chart

CHART 92

To what factors should I pay particular attention in regard to my job?

1. organization
2. planning
3. development
4. efficiency
5. objectivity
6. growth
7. research
8. costs/gain
9. conflict/politics
10. evaluation
11. expenses/gain
12. profiling
13. communication
14. teamwork
15. not on this chart

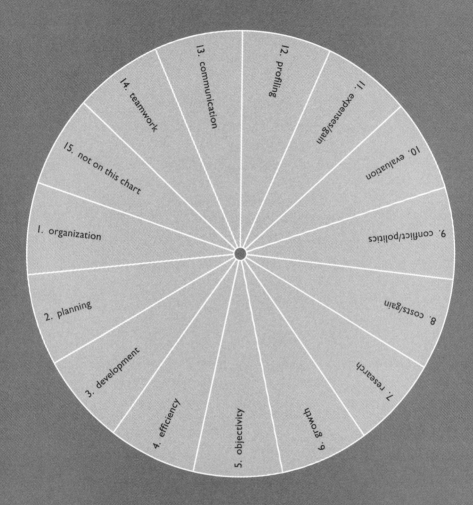

13. communication
12. profiling
14. teamwork
11. expenses/gain
15. not on this chart
10. evaluation
1. organization
9. conflict/politics
2. planning
8. costs/gain
3. development
7. research
4. efficiency
5. objectivity
6. growth

To what factors should I pay particular attention in regard to my job?

CHART 93

What talents/abilities/qualities do I have?

1. communication gifts
2. independence
3. good intellectual grasp
4. planning and organizational skills
5. collaboration
6. creativity
7. scientific research
8. responsibility
9. intuition
10. charm
11. editorial work
12. artistic ability
13. stability
14. musical talents
15. not on this chart

SEE ALSO PENDULUM CHARTS 83, 84, 94

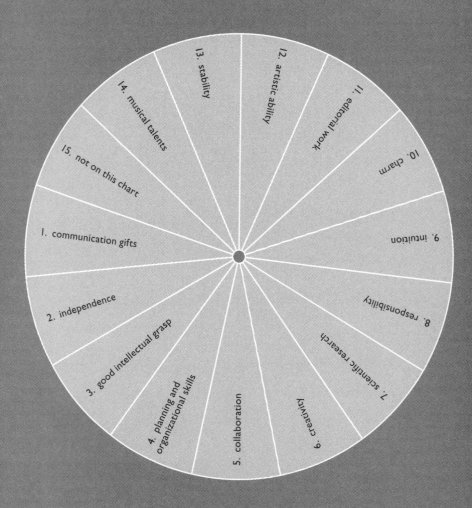

What talents/abilities/qualities do I have?

CHART 94

I foster my talent above all _____.

1. through my work/my job
2. through the right education
3. by keeping eyes and ears open
4. by playing
5. by surrounding myself with other . . .
6. by occupying myself with one topic
7. by using it very fully
8. by gathering new experience
9. through regular practicing
10. by giving myself difficult tasks
11. by putting myself in stressful . . .
12. by taking a lot of time for myself
13. by concentrating on one single goal
14. by taking good advice to heart
15. not on this chart

SEE ALSO PENDULUM CHARTS 83, 84, 93

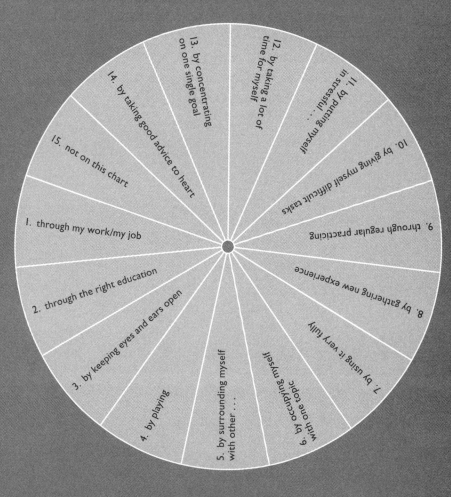

12. by taking a lot of time for myself

11. by putting myself in stressful …

10. by giving myself difficult tasks

9. through regular practicing

8. by gathering new experience

7. by using it very fully

6. by occupying myself with one topic

5. by surrounding myself with other …

4. by playing

3. by keeping eyes and ears open

2. through the right education

1. through my work/my job

15. not on this chart

14. by taking good advice to heart

13. by concentrating on one single goal

I foster my talent above all _____

CHART 95

Friendship is important to me because:

1. I am a social person
2. I like to tell stories
3. I like to listen to the stories of others
4. it is a great support to me
5. I have a lot of fun
6. I like to go out with others
7. I get a lot of new ideas and impulses
8. I want to share my feelings
9. I am curious about the opinion . . .
10. I don't like to be lonely
11. I like to have people around me
12. I need feedback
13. I want to share my experiences
14. I want to be a good friend
15. not on this chart

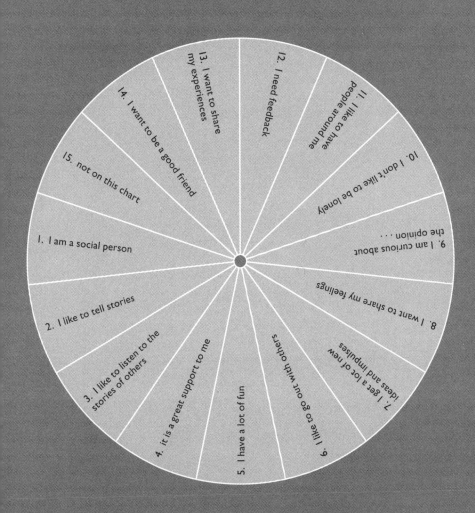

Friendship is important to me because:

1. I am a social person
2. I like to tell stories
3. I like to listen to the stories of others
4. it is a great support to me
5. I have a lot of fun
6. I like to go out with others
7. I get a lot of new ideas and impulses
8. I want to share my feelings
9. I am curious about the opinion . . .
10. I don't like to be lonely
11. I like to have people around me
12. I need feedback
13. I want to share my experiences
14. I want to be a good friend
15. not on this chart

CHART 96

My best male friend is my _____.

1. husband
2. buddy
3. father
4. brother
5. uncle
6. cousin
7. son
8. fellow student
9. colleague
10. companion/business partner
11. housemate/roommate
12. neighbor
13. pet
14. lover
15. not on this chart

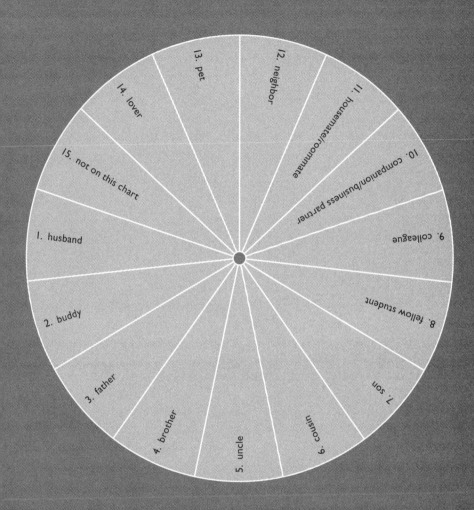

1. husband
2. buddy
3. father
4. brother
5. uncle
6. cousin
7. son
8. fellow student
9. colleague
10. companion/business partner
11. housemate/roommate
12. neighbor
13. pet
14. lover
15. not on this chart

My best male friend is my _____.

CHART 97

My best female friend is my _____.

1. wife
2. girlfriend
3. mother
4. sister
5. aunt
6. cousin
7. daughter
8. fellow student
9. co-worker
10. companion/business partner
11. housemate/roommate
12. neighbor
13. pet
14. lover
15. not on this chart

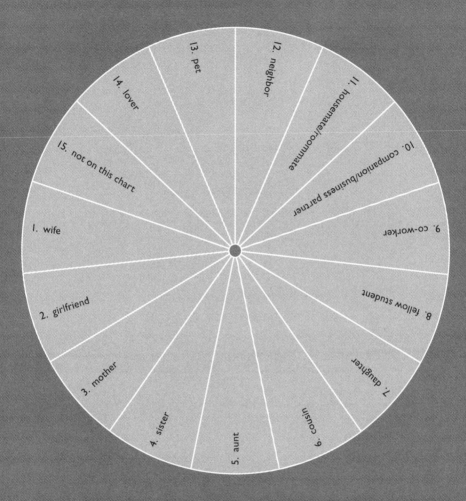

13. pet
12. neighbor
14. lover
11. housemate/roommate
10. companion/business partner
15. not on this chart
9. co-worker
1. wife
2. girlfriend
8. fellow student
3. mother
7. daughter
4. sister
6. cousin
5. aunt

My best female friend is my _____.

CHART 98

Which feature or characteristic of my partner do I find most attractive?

1. unconditional love
2. erotic attraction
3. humor
4. intelligence
5. reliability
6. honesty
7. mother/father figure
8. financial security
9. status
10. compatibility
11. soul mates
12. warmth
13. enthusiasm
14. perseverance
15. curiosity
16. enjoyment of life
17. balance
18. adventurousness
19. idealism
20. looks
21. optimism
22. creativity
23. athletic ability
24. passion
25. not on this chart

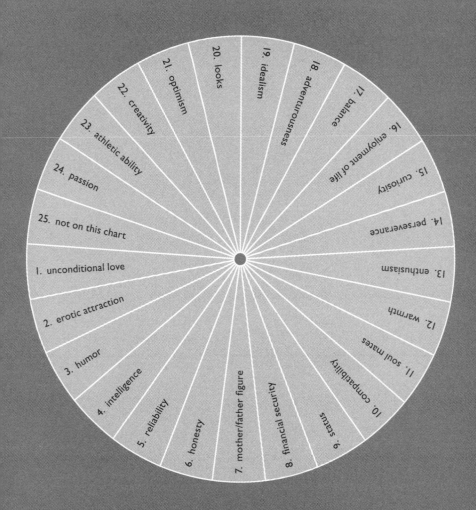

*Which feature or characteristic of my partner
do I find most attractive?*

CHART 99

To me, my current relationship means _____.

1. I have found my soul mate
2. I am getting to know myself better
3. I can share my life
4. I have found peace and quiet
5. I can make a new beginning
6. I can dare to be egoistical
7. I am learning to accept myself
8. I am learning to accept my partner
9. I can sacrifice myself
10. I can start a family
11. I can be independent
12. my life has changed drastically
13. a phase of contemplation
14. does not apply
15. not on this chart

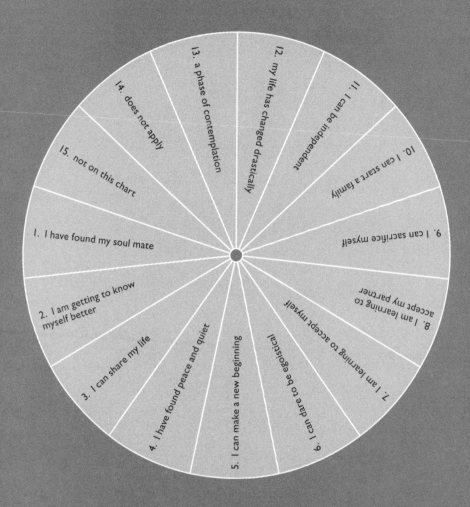

1. I have found my soul mate
2. I am getting to know myself better
3. I can share my life
4. I have found peace and quiet
5. I can make a new beginning
6. I can dare to be egoistical
7. I am learning to accept myself
8. I am learning to accept my partner
9. I can sacrifice myself
10. I can start a family
11. I can be independent
12. my life has changed drastically
13. a phase of contemplation
14. does not apply
15. not on this chart

To me, my current relationship means _____.

CHART 100

The best way for me to relax is _____.

1. lying lazily on the couch
2. listening to music or making music
3. taking part in sports
4. solving difficult problems
5. having fun with others
6. taking a long walk
7. caring for my pet
8. making myself a present
9. cooking plenty of food
10. working in the garden
11. watching television
12. eating in a restaurant
13. going on an excursion
14. helping a friend
15. not on this chart

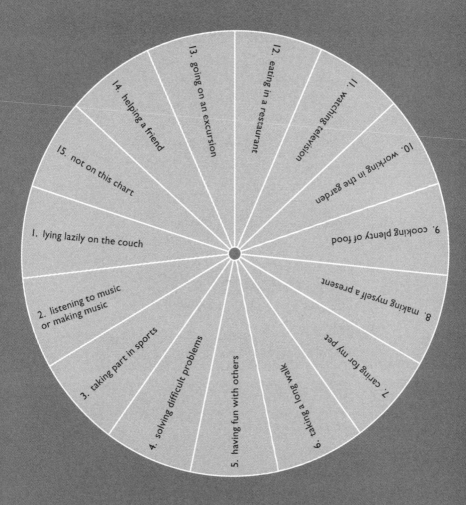

The best way for me to relax is _____.

1. lying lazily on the couch
2. listening to music or making music
3. taking part in sports
4. solving difficult problems
5. having fun with others
6. taking a long walk
7. caring for my pet
8. making myself a present
9. cooking plenty of food
10. working in the garden
11. watching television
12. eating in a restaurant
13. going on an excursion
14. helping a friend
15. not on this chart

CHART 101

I get rid of my bad moods—at home—best if _____.

1. I listen to my favorite music
2. I do something "useful"
3. I call my best friend
4. I write a letter
5. I clean up
6. I listen to music and sing or dance
7. I make fun of my roommate
8. I do nothing at all
9. I cry loudly or scream
10. I am very impolite
11. I meditate
12. I have a good talk with myself
13. I read a thick book
14. I take a bubble bath
15. not on this chart

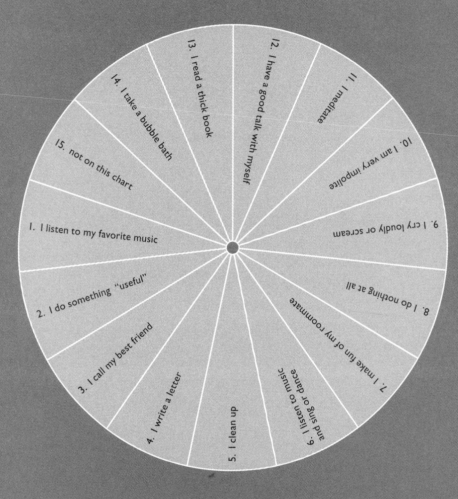

13. I read a thick book

12. I have a good talk with myself

11. I meditate

14. I take a bubble bath

10. I am very impolite

15. not on this chart

9. I cry loudly or scream

1. I listen to my favorite music

8. I do nothing at all

2. I do something "useful"

7. I make fun of my roommate

3. I call my best friend

6. I listen to music and sing or dance

4. I write a letter

5. I clean up

I get rid of my bad moods—at home—best if _____.

CHART 102

When I play hooky I prefer to do the following:

1. drive around in my car
2. visit a restaurant
3. order the biggest sundae
4. go on a shopping trip
5. sit for hours at a sunny café
6. visit a museum
7. spontaneously visit my friends
8. dream the time away
9. accept an invitation spontaneously
10. at last finish that thick book
11. watch that very long movie
12. take a stroll in nature
13. pretend that I'm not playing hooky
14. convince others to play hooky too
15. not on this chart

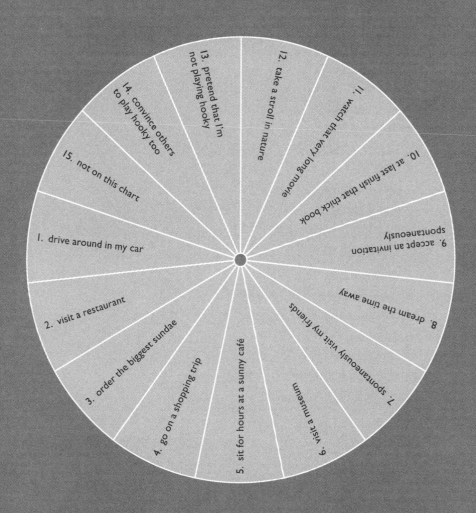

1. drive around in my car
2. visit a restaurant
3. order the biggest sundae
4. go on a shopping trip
5. sit for hours at a sunny café
6. visit a museum
7. spontaneously visit my friends
8. dream the time away
9. accept an invitation spontaneously
10. at last finish that thick book
11. watch that very long movie
12. take a stroll in nature
13. pretend that I'm not playing hooky
14. convince others to play hooky too
15. not on this chart

When I play hooky I prefer to do the following:

CHART 103

What music has a positive influence on me?

1. classical music
2. cool jazz
3. rock and roll
4. blues
5. pop (general)
6. modern (general)
7. country/ western
8. oriental folk music
9. occidental folk music
10. new age
11. dixieland
12. religious music (e.g. gospel)
13. reggae
14. hip hop
15. show music
16. big band music
17. fusion
18. easy listening
19. ballet music
20. opera
21. operetta
22. a capella
23. vocals
24. instrumental music
25. not on this chart

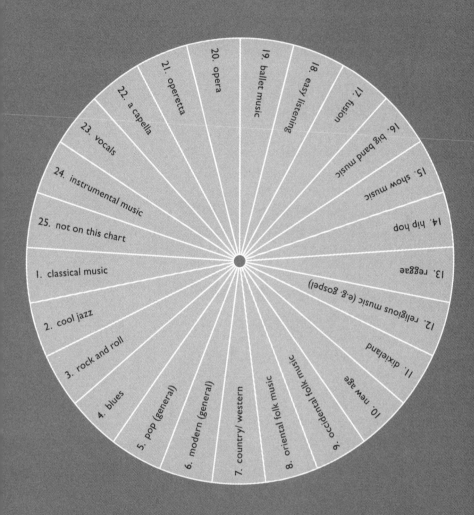

20. opera
21. operetta
22. a capella
23. vocals
24. instrumental music
25. not on this chart
1. classical music
2. cool jazz
3. rock and roll
4. blues
5. pop (general)
6. modern (general)
7. country/ western
8. oriental folk music
9. occidental folk music
10. new age
11. dixieland
12. religious music (e.g. gospel)
13. reggae
14. hip hop
15. show music
16. big band music
17. fusion
18. easy listening
19. ballet music

What music has a positive influence on me?

CHART 104

What kind of vacation (holiday destination) suits me well?

1. safari with camera
2. foreign travel
3. does not matter as long as it is far . . .
4. solitude
5. hiking in the mountains
6. sailing
7. skiing
8. hiking
9. biking
10. horseback riding
11. keywords: sun, ocean, beach
12. keywords: lazy, luxurious, good food
13. keywords: new experience . . .
14. keyword: adventure
15. fishing
16. survivor training
17. camping
18. white water rafting/kayaking
19. cruise
20. trekking through the jungle
21. cultural group trip
22. adventurous group trip
23. hiking alone through nature
24. rock or mountain climbing
25. not on this chart

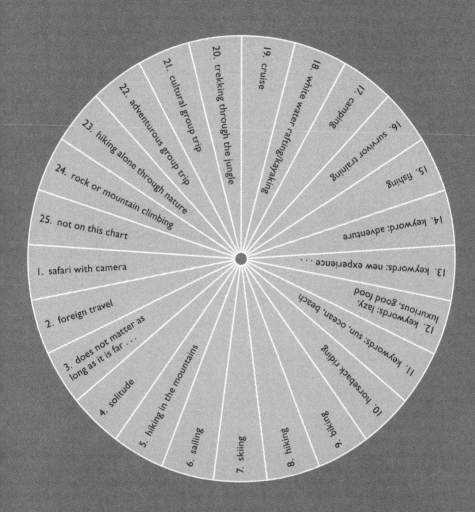

What kind of vacation (holiday destination) suits me well?

The following options appear around the wheel:

- 1. safari with camera
- 2. foreign travel
- 3. does not matter as long as it is far . . .
- 4. solitude
- 5. hiking in the mountains
- 6. sailing
- 7. skiing
- 8. hiking
- 9. biking
- 10. horseback riding
- 11. keywords: sun, ocean, beach
- 12. keywords: lazy, luxurious, good food
- 13. keywords: new experience . . .
- 14. keyword: adventure
- 15. fishing
- 16. survivor training
- 17. camping
- 18. white water rafting/kayaking
- 19. cruise
- 20. trekking through the jungle
- 21. cultural group trip
- 22. adventurous group trip
- 23. hiking alone through nature
- 24. rock or mountain climbing
- 25. not on this chart

CHART 105

What sport suits me best?

1. biking
2. hiking
3. "extreme" sports
4. canoeing (in wild water)
5. soccer
6. ball games
7. hockey/ice hockey
8. tennis, badminton
9. running, athletics, track
10. weight training
11. energy sports set to music
12. polo/water polo
13. martial arts
14. rugby/lacrosse
15. long-distance sports
16. gymnastics, acrobatics, etc.
17. golf
18. swimming
19. synchronized swimming or diving
20. in-line skating
21. ice skating
22. skiing
23. fencing
24. horseback riding
25. not on this chart

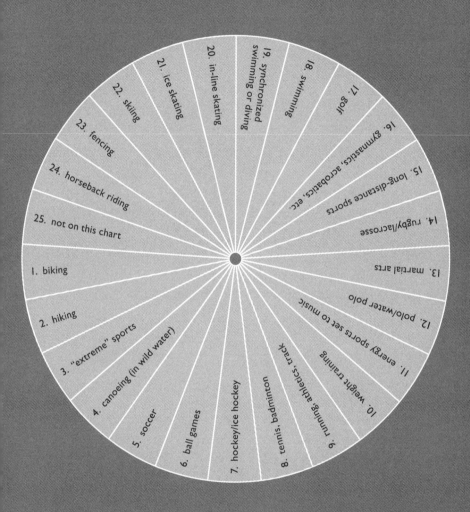

19. synchronized swimming or diving
18. swimming
17. golf
16. gymnastics, acrobatics, etc.
15. long-distance sports
14. rugby/lacrosse
13. martial arts
12. polo/water polo
11. energy sports set to music
10. weight training
9. running, athletics, track
8. tennis, badminton
7. hockey/ice hockey
6. ball games
5. soccer
4. canoeing (in wild water)
3. "extreme" sports
2. hiking
1. biking
25. not on this chart
24. horseback riding
23. fencing
22. skiing
21. ice skating
20. in-line skating

What sport suits me best?

CHART 106

At what social games do I shine?

1. simple board games
2. strategy board games
3. Battleship
4. word games
5. games that stimulate the imagination
6. games that require knowledge of facts
7. strategic games
8. memory games
9. gambling games
10. card games
11. Dungeons and Dragons
12. games of skill, relay races
13. narrating a "continuing story"
14. charades
15. not on this chart

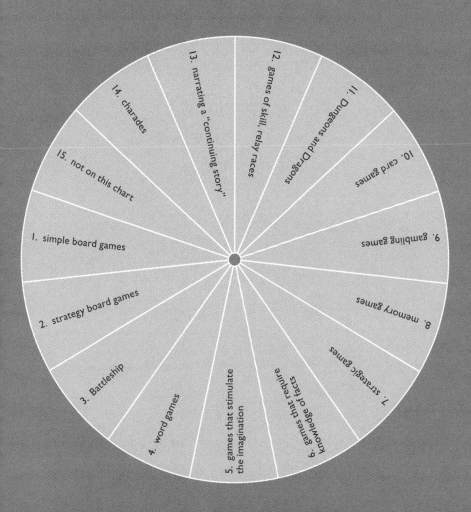

At what social games do I shine?

1. simple board games
2. strategy board games
3. Battleship
4. word games
5. games that stimulate the imagination
6. games that require knowledge of facts
7. strategic games
8. memory games
9. gambling games
10. card games
11. Dungeons and Dragons
12. games of skill, relay races
13. narrating a "continuing story"
14. charades
15. not on this chart

CHART 107

What is most important to me in my environment?

1. peace
2. harmony
3. silence
4. fresh air
5. a lot of space
6. security
7. sunlight
8. order
9. comfort
10. warmth
11. privacy
12. luxury
13. simplicity
14. style
15. not on this chart

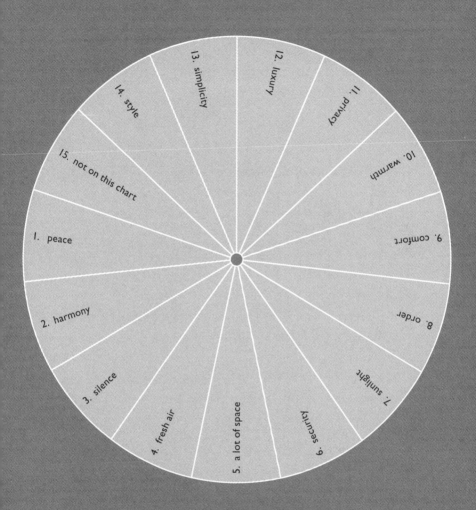

1. peace
2. harmony
3. silence
4. fresh air
5. a lot of space
6. security
7. sunlight
8. order
9. comfort
10. warmth
11. privacy
12. luxury
13. simplicity
14. style
15. not on this chart

What is most important to me in my environment?

CHART 108

*What materials in my immediate surroundings have
a positive affect on me?*

1. hardwood
2. bamboo
3. cork
4. sisal
5. straw or carpet-of-rice straw
6. glass
7. paper/cardboard
8. wool
9. cotton
10. precious metals
11. plastics
12. aluminum
13. Plexiglas
14. ceramic
15. linoleum
16. marble
17. high-grade steel
18. copper
19. chrome
20. leather
21. vinyl
22. terrazzo
23. fiberboard
24. jute
25. not on this chart

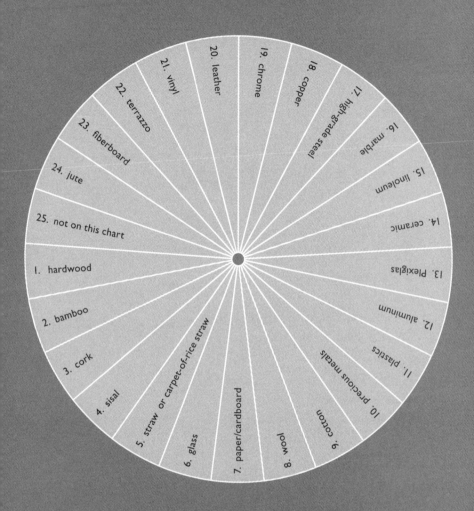

*What materials in my immediate surroundings
have a positive affect on me?*

CHART 109

What materials in my immediate surroundings should I avoid?

1. hardwood
2. bamboo
3. cork
4. sisal
5. straw or carpet-of-rice straw
6. glass
7. paper/cardboard
8. wool
9. cotton
10. precious metals
11. plastics
12. aluminum
13. Plexiglas
14. ceramic
15. linoleum
16. marble
17. high-grade steel
18. copper
19. chrome
20. leather
21. vinyl
22. terrazzo
23. fiberboard
24. jute
25. not on this chart

SEE ALSO PENDULUM CHARTS 12, 31, 32, 55, 119

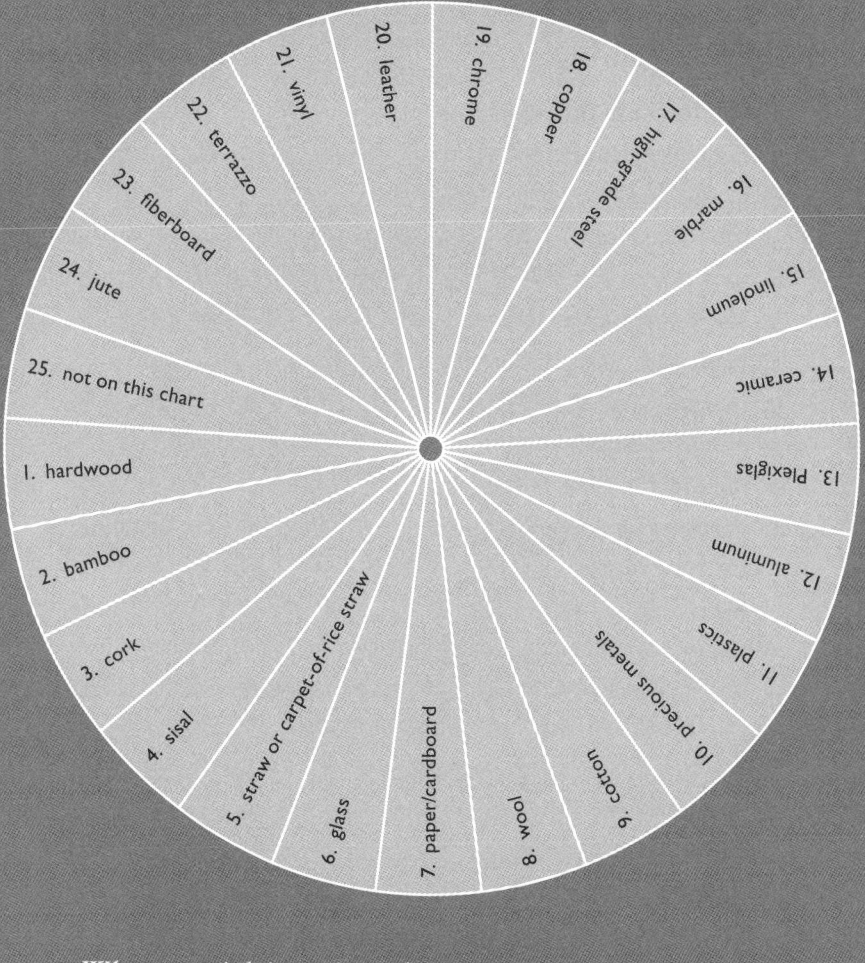

1. hardwood
2. bamboo
3. cork
4. sisal
5. straw or carpet-of-rice straw
6. glass
7. paper/cardboard
8. wool
9. cotton
10. precious metals
11. plastics
12. aluminum
13. Plexiglas
14. ceramic
15. linoleum
16. marble
17. high-grade steel
18. copper
19. chrome
20. leather
21. vinyl
22. terrazzo
23. fiberboard
24. jute
25. not on this chart

What materials in my immediate surroundings should I avoid?

CHART 110

What kind of home suits me best?

1. apartment in the heart of a big city
2. apartment in the suburbs
3. luxury penthouse
4. garage apartment
5. suburban home
6. part of a duplex
7. small hideaway in the country
8. large farmhouse in the country
9. bungalow
10. renovated loft
11. historic building
12. basement apartment
13. trailer/camper
14. houseboat
15. not on this chart

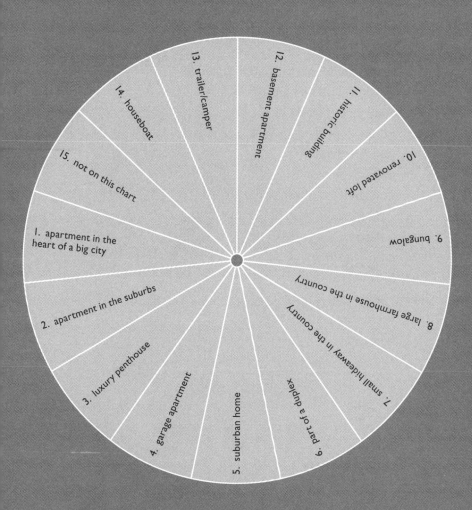

1. apartment in the heart of a big city
2. apartment in the suburbs
3. luxury penthouse
4. garage apartment
5. suburban home
6. part of a duplex
7. small hideaway in the country
8. large farmhouse in the country
9. bungalow
10. renovated loft
11. historic building
12. basement apartment
13. trailer/camper
14. houseboat
15. not on this chart

What kind of home suits me best?

CHART III

What kind of home would be difficult for me to live in?

1. apartment in the heart of a big city
2. apartment in the suburbs
3. luxury penthouse
4. garage apartment
5. suburban home
6. part of a duplex
7. small hideaway in the country
8. large farmhouse in the country
9. bungalow
10. renovated loft
11. historical building
12. basement apartment
13. trailer/camper
14. houseboat
15. not on this chart

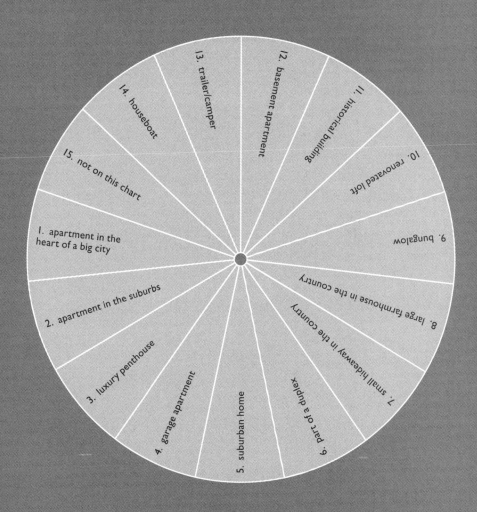

1. apartment in the heart of a big city
2. apartment in the suburbs
3. luxury penthouse
4. garage apartment
5. suburban home
6. part of a duplex
7. small hideaway in the country
8. large farmhouse in the country
9. bungalow
10. renovated loft
11. historical building
12. basement apartment
13. trailer/camper
14. houseboat
15. not on this chart

What kind of home would be difficult for me to live in?

CHART 112

Which part of my home needs special attention—#1?

1. walls
2. floors
3. ceilings
4. roof
5. attic
6. windows
7. doors
8. air conditioning
9. heating
10. electrical wires and supplies
11. gas lines
12. water pipes and faucets
13. drains, waste pipes
14. insulation
15. not on this chart

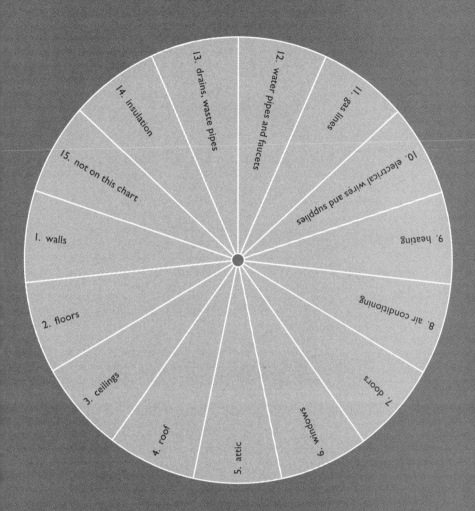

Which part of my home needs special attention—#1?

CHART 113

Which part of my home needs special attention—#2?

1. living room
2. dining room
3. bedroom
4. study or office
5. hobby- or playroom
6. children's room
7. bathroom
8. closets
9. basement
10. foyer
11. hallway(s)
12. kitchen
13. laundry room
14. staircase
15. not on this chart

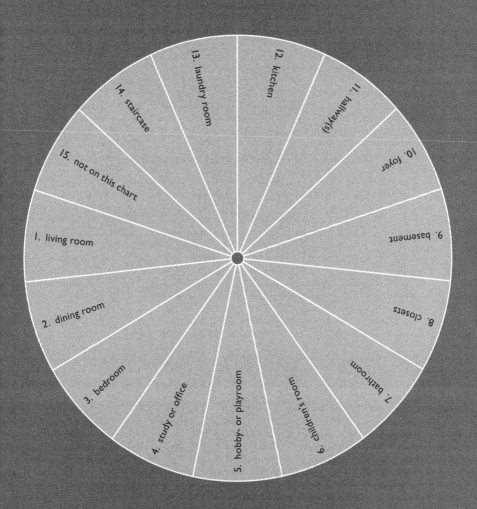

12. kitchen

11. hallway(s)

13. laundry room

10. foyer

14. staircase

9. basement

15. not on this chart

1. living room

8. closets

2. dining room

7. bathroom

3. bedroom

6. children's room

4. study or office

5. hobby- or playroom

Which part of my home needs special attention—#2?

CHART 114

What kind of room suits me best?

1. small, comfortable room
2. large, comfortable room
3. small, cozy room
4. small, sparsely furnished room
5. large, sparsely furnished room
6. small, very sunny room
7. large, very sunny room
8. small room with beautiful view
9. large room with beautiful view
10. room with all modern conveniences
11. room in which I can receive friends
12. room with lots of bookcases
13. room in which my stereo is the focus
14. room in which television . . .
15. not on this chart

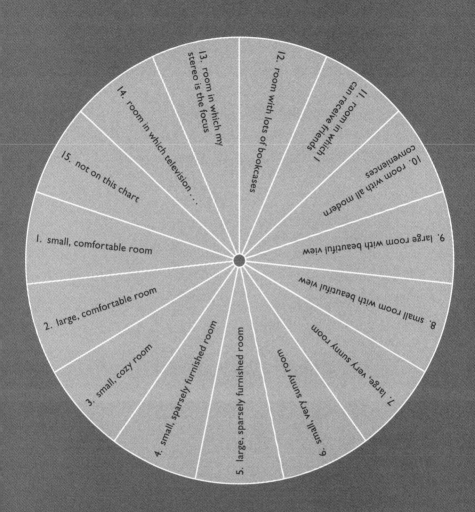

What kind of room suits me best?

1. small, comfortable room
2. large, comfortable room
3. small, cozy room
4. small, sparsely furnished room
5. large, sparsely furnished room
6. small, very sunny room
7. large, very sunny room
8. small room with beautiful view
9. large room with beautiful view
10. room with all modern conveniences
11. room in which I can receive friends
12. room with lots of bookcases
13. room in which my stereo is the focus
14. room in which television...
15. not on this chart

CHART 115

In what kind of room do I feel uncomfortable?

1. small room with too much furniture
2. large room with too much furniture
3. small room with too little furniture
4. large room with too little furniture
5. very light room
6. very dark room
7. room without a view
8. room with a beautiful view
9. room that is easy to peek into
10. messy room
11. too tidy a room
12. formal room
13. rustic room
14. living room with various styles
15. not on this chart

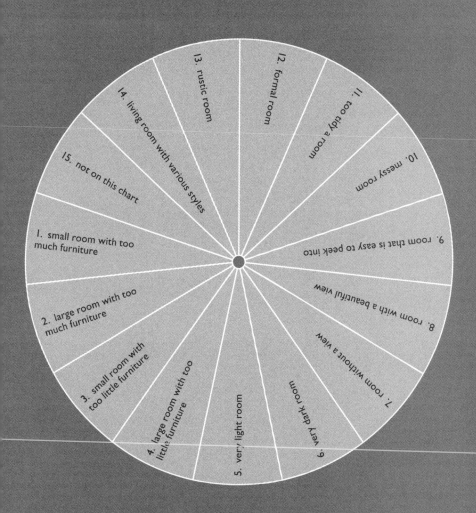

In what kind of room do I feel uncomfortable?

CHART 116

What kind of workplace suits me best?

1. small office with desk and phone
2. large office shared by two people
3. home office
4. newsroom
5. outdoors
6. retail shop
7. small office with great view
8. large office with great view
9. workshop
10. garage
11. bank
12. hospital
13. theatre
14. studio
15. not on this chart

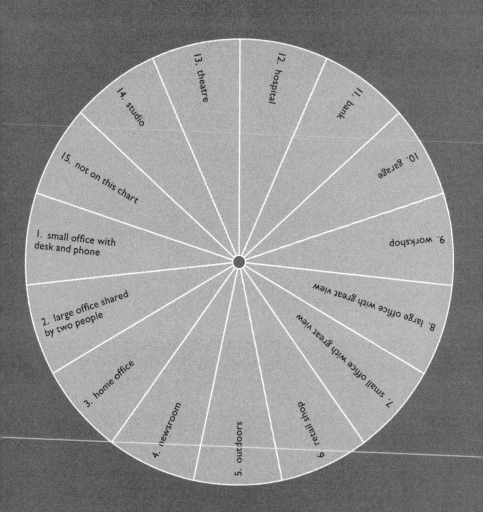

1. small office with desk and phone
2. large office shared by two people
3. home office
4. newsroom
5. outdoors
6. retail shop
7. small office with great view
8. large office with great view
9. workshop
10. garage
11. bank
12. hospital
13. theatre
14. studio
15. not on this chart

What kind of workplace suits me best?

CHART 117

What kind of workplace should I avoid?

1. small office with desk and phone
2. large office shared by two people
3. home office
4. newsroom
5. outdoors
6. retail shop
7. small office with great view
8. large office with great view
9. workshop
10. garage
11. bank
12. hospital
13. theatre
14. studio
15. not on this chart

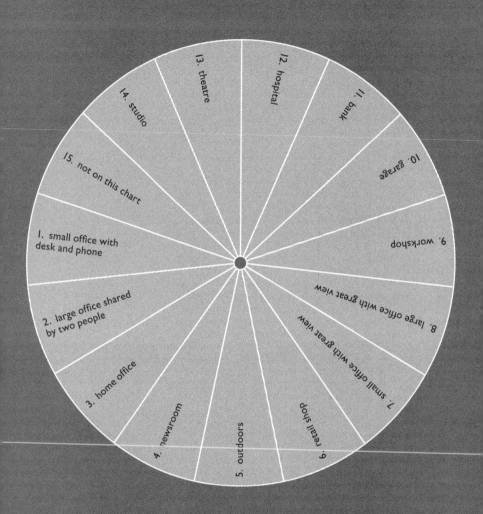

14. studio

13. theatre

12. hospital

11. bank

10. garage

15. not on this chart

9. workshop

1. small office with desk and phone

8. large office with great view

2. large office shared by two people

7. small office with great view

3. home office

6. retail shop

4. newsroom

5. outdoors

What kind of workplace should I avoid?

CHART 118

What indoor plants have a positive influence on me?

1. rubber plant
2. ivy
3. date palm
4. African violet
5. fern
6. bromeliad
7. chrysanthemum
8. philodendron
9. dieffenbachia
10. snake plant
11. cactus
12. bamboo
13. spider plant
14. flamingo flower
15. poinsettia
16. azalea
17. prayer plant
18. aloe vera
19. geranium
20. palm
21. begonia
22. dragon tree
23. jade plant
24. bonsai
25. not on this chart

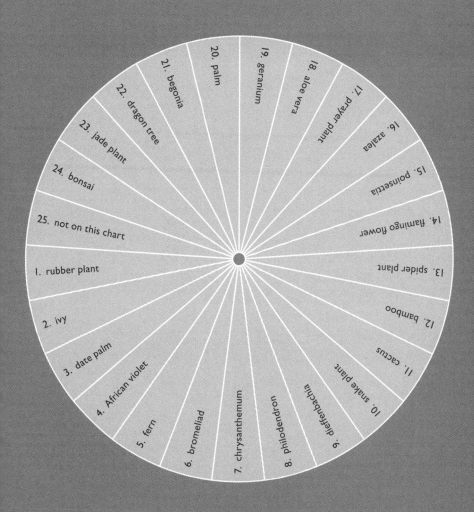

20. palm
21. begonia
22. dragon tree
23. jade plant
24. bonsai
25. not on this chart
1. rubber plant
2. ivy
3. date palm
4. African violet
5. fern
6. bromeliad
7. chrysanthemum
8. philodendron
9. dieffenbachia
10. snake plant
11. cactus
12. bamboo
13. spider plant
14. flamingo flower
15. poinsettia
16. azalea
17. prayer plant
18. aloe vera
19. geranium

What indoor plants have a positive influence on me?

CHART 119

What indoor plants would it be better for me to avoid?

1. rubber plant
2. ivy
3. date palm
4. African violet
5. fern
6. bromeliad
7. chrysanthemum
8. philodendron
9. dieffenbachia
10. snake plant
11. cactus
12. bamboo
13. spider plant
14. flamingo flower
15. poinsettia or Christmas rose
16. azalea
17. prayer plant
18. aloe vera
19. geranium
20. palm
21. begonia
22. dragon tree
23. jade plant
24. bonsai
25. not on this chart

SEE ALSO PENDULUM CHARTS 12, 34, 35, 117

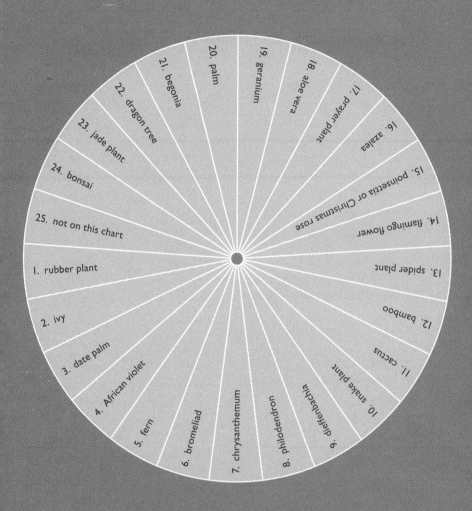

1. rubber plant
2. ivy
3. date palm
4. African violet
5. fern
6. bromeliad
7. chrysanthemum
8. philodendron
9. dieffenbachia
10. snake plant
11. cactus
12. bamboo
13. spider plant
14. flamingo flower
15. poinsettia or Christmas rose
16. azalea
17. prayer plant
18. aloe vera
19. geranium
20. palm
21. begonia
22. dragon tree
23. jade plant
24. bonsai
25. not on this chart

What indoor plants would it be better for me to avoid?

CHART 120

What flower should I plant in my garden—#1?

1. rose
2. dahlia
3. violet
4. marigold
5. clematis
6. pansy
7. passionflower
8. geranium
9. hydrangea
10. iris
11. petunia
12. lily-of-the-valley
13. poppy
14. nasturtium
15. peony
16. rhododendron
17. salvia
18. larkspur
19. hollyhock
20. morning glory
21. zinnia
22. foxglove
23. snapdragon
24. bleeding heart
25. not on this chart

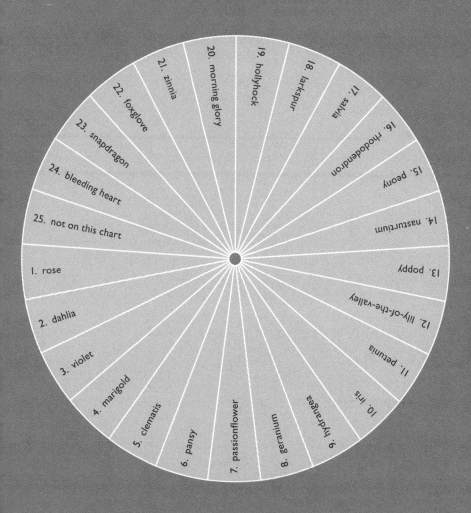

21. zinnia
22. foxglove
23. snapdragon
24. bleeding heart
25. not on this chart
1. rose
2. dahlia
3. violet
4. marigold
5. clematis
6. pansy
7. passionflower
8. geranium
9. hydrangea
10. iris
11. petunia
12. lily-of-the-valley
13. poppy
14. nasturtium
15. peony
16. rhododendron
17. salvia
18. larkspur
19. hollyhock
20. morning glory

What flower should I plant in my garden—#1?

CHART 121

What flower should I plant in my garden—#2?

1. sweet pea
2. anemone
3. fuschia
4. sweet william
5. aster
6. fern
7. lilac
8. delphinium
9. tulip
10. hyacinth
11. narcissus
12. crocus
13. campanula
14. daffodil
15. alyssum
16. carnation
17. sunflower
18. lily
19. gladiolus
20. baby's breath
21. primula plant
22. Easter lily
23. chrysanthemum
24. impatiens
25. not on this chart

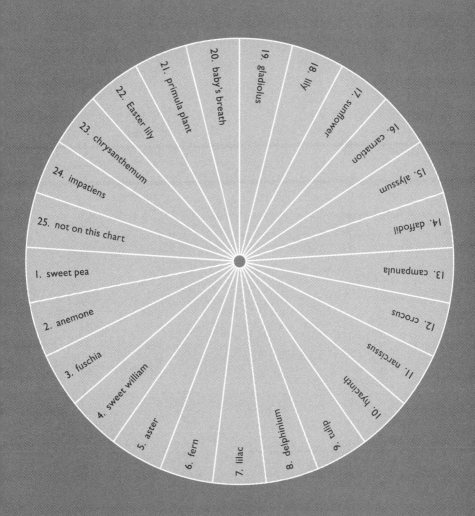

What flower should I plant in my garden—#2?

CHART 122

What wild plant has a positive influence on me—#1?

1. lupine
2. evening primrose
3. hyssop
4. columbine
5. milkweed
6. butterflyweed
7. indigo
8. wild senna
9. coreopsis
10. shooting star
11. boneset
12. clover
13. sneezeweed
14. cornflower
15. black-eyed Susan
16. rattlesnake master
17. wild rose
18. wild onion
19. flowering spurge
20. prairie cinquefoil
21. wild quinine
22. mountain mint
23. cardinal flower
24. smooth penstemon
25. not on this chart

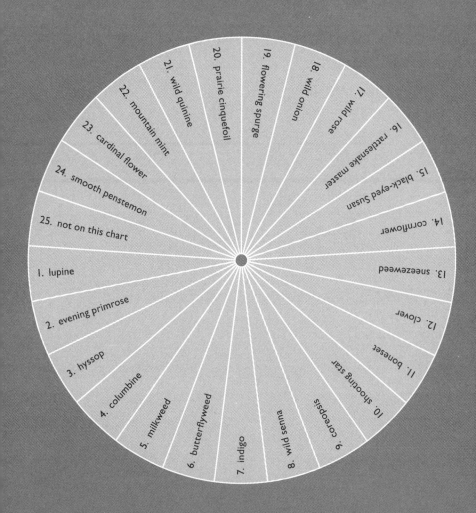

What wild plant has a positive influence on me—#1?

Wheel segments (clockwise):

- 19. flowering spurge
- 18. wild onion
- 17. wild rose
- 16. rattlesnake master
- 15. black-eyed Susan
- 14. cornflower
- 13. sneezeweed
- 12. clover
- 11. boneset
- 10. shooting star
- 9. coreopsis
- 8. wild senna
- 7. indigo
- 6. butterflyweed
- 5. milkweed
- 4. columbine
- 3. hyssop
- 2. evening primrose
- 1. lupine
- 25. not on this chart
- 24. smooth penstemon
- 23. cardinal flower
- 22. mountain mint
- 21. wild quinine
- 20. prairie cinquefoil

CHART 123

What wild plant has a positive influence on me—#2?

1. beardtongue
2. meadow blazingstar
3. great blue lobelia
4. sage
5. royal catchfly
6. spiderwort
7. blue vervain
8. Canada milk vetch
9. Jacob's ladder
10. false dragonhead
11. culver's root
12. golden alexander
13. Queen Anne's lace
14. calendula
15. chicory
16. ox eye daisy
17. cosmos
18. foxglove
19. Indian blanket
20. candytuft
21. flax
22. bluebonnet
23. forget-me-not
24. bluebell
25. not on this chart

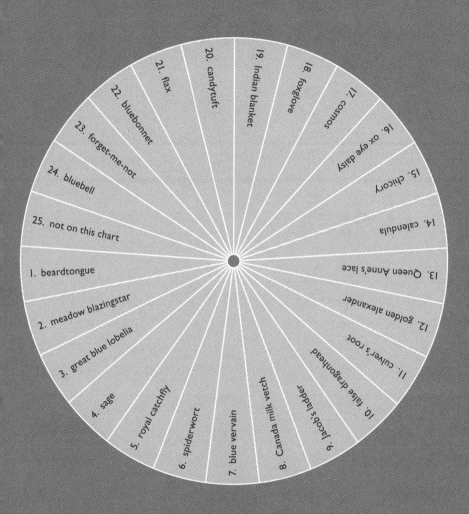

What wild plant has a positive influence on me—#2?

CHART 124

What kind of garden suits me best?

1. formal garden
2. Japanese garden
3. Zen garden
4. container garden
5. wild garden with sun and shade
6. window sill garden
7. water garden
8. terrace garden
9. patio garden
10. herb garden
11. vegetable garden
12. kitchen garden
13. cottage garden
14. bird sanctuary
15. not on this chart

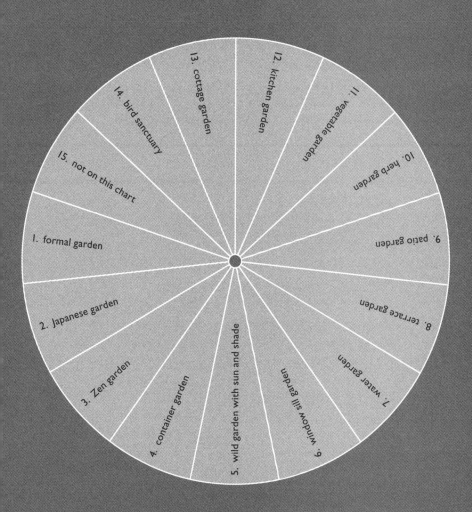

What kind of garden suits me best?

1. formal garden
2. Japanese garden
3. Zen garden
4. container garden
5. wild garden with sun and shade
6. window sill garden
7. water garden
8. terrace garden
9. patio garden
10. herb garden
11. vegetable garden
12. kitchen garden
13. cottage garden
14. bird sanctuary
15. not on this chart

CHART 125

What kind of "recreation area" do I find most appealing?

1. my own garden
2. park in my immediate vicinity
3. city park
4. national park or hiking area
5. forest
6. dunes
7. beach
8. wetlands
9. desert
10. mountain lookout
11. lakeside
12. riverbank
13. backyard hammock
14. terrace shadowed by trees
15. not on this chart

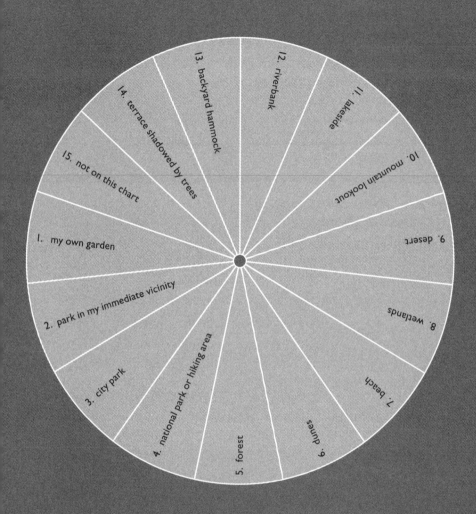

What kind of "recreation area" do I find most appealing?

1. my own garden
2. park in my immediate vicinity
3. city park
4. national park or hiking area
5. forest
6. dunes
7. beach
8. wetlands
9. desert
10. mountain lookout
11. lakeside
12. riverbank
13. backyard hammock
14. terrace shadowed by trees
15. not on this chart

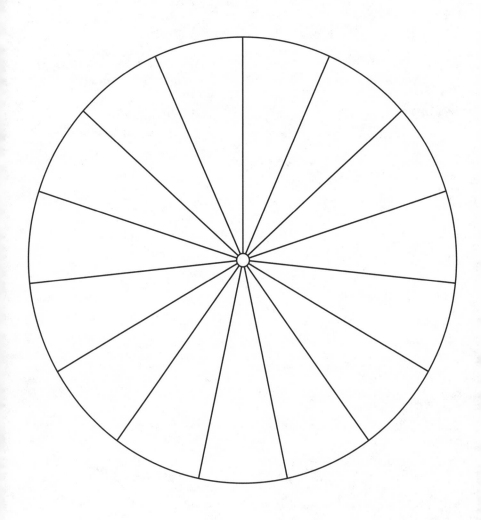

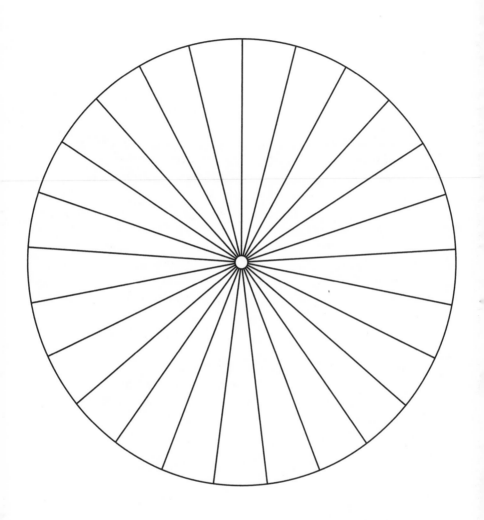

Index